Caring Architecture

Caring Architecture:

Institutions and Relational Practices

Edited by

Catharina Nord and Ebba Högström

Cambridge
Scholars
Publishing

Caring Architecture: Institutions and Relational Practices

Edited by Catharina Nord and Ebba Högström

This book first published 2017

Cambridge Scholars Publishing

Lady Stephenson Library, Newcastle upon Tyne, NE6 2PA, UK

British Library Cataloguing in Publication Data
A catalogue record for this book is available from the British Library

ISBN (10): 1-4438-9896-1
ISBN (13): 978-1-4438-9896-6

TABLE OF CONTENTS

LIST OF ILLUSTRATIONS

Acknowledgements

This book is based on a session at the RGS-IBG Annual International Conference, which was held in London in August, 2014. We would like to thank Cambridge Scholars Publishing for inviting us to develop the themes pursued in that session into a book. We offer our thanks in particular to Victoria Carruthers, who patiently waited for us to finalise the manuscript and has supported us in meeting all challenges which arose whilst putting together this volume.

Special thanks go to our contributors for their commitment and endurance, and for responding to our suggestions and proposals with such a positive spirit. Thank you all. We would like to offer our gratitude to Gunnar Olsson for accepting our invitation to participate in a scholarly dialogue with Martin Gren. We are very honoured to have the voice of such an eminent scholar in Swedish geographical research present in this publication.

Our sincere thanks also go to our colleagues who provided comments and assisted in reviewing the first version of the texts in this anthology. Their contribution improved the scientific quality of the different chapters substantially. In alphabetical order, we therefore thank: Andrew Byerley, Cameron Duff, Catharina Gabrielsson, Martin Gren, Jonathan Metzger, Christer Persson, Meike Schalk, Ola Söderström and Moa Tunström.

We also wish to acknowledge the generosity of Mrs. Arabella M. R. Hobson in granting us permission on behalf of the Godfrey family to use the drawing of Morden college drafted by her grandfather, Walter H. Godfrey.

We also want to thank Helen Runting for editing services and linguistic advice.

Finally, thanks go to Prof. Abdellah Abarkan, Head of Department of Spatial Planning at Blekinge Institute of Technology for providing financial support for this project, and also to the doctoral students at the National Institute for the Study of Ageing and Later Life (NISAL) at Linköping University who provided valuable comments in relation to Catharina Nord's chapter.

COMMENTARY I

BETWEEN CARING AND ARCHITECTURE

GUNNAR OLSSON AND MARTIN GREN

MG: What is the first thing that pops up in your mind when you hear the expression "caring architecture"?

GO: That it is a falsity. Any architecture that is intentional is a way of forming other people, so I immediately sense an inevitable closeness between caring architecture and imprisoning architecture.

MG: So, architecture is about intentionally forming other people by physical structures?

GO: Yes, and you can have different intentions when you are forming the physical structures, but you are making a great mistake if you forget that the very point of building is to shape other people's lives. It can be life in prison, in the caring home for the elderly, or in the living room where we now are sitting. How you do this forming obviously varies, but the fundamental idea is that by structuring spatial space you are simultaneously structuring people.

MG: Regardless of what kind of architecture we are talking about it is always intimately linked to relationships of power.

GO: Yes, architecture itself is very much steeped in power since its very essence is to form or delimit people's behaviour. It is always about power-relations, about moving from physical infrastructure, like the concrete walls in front of you and me, into our malleable minds.

MG: In that sense, there is a straight line to be drawn from the architect to the politician.

GO: Well, there is no real modern politician who does not know that the very point of politics is to form people's minds. A serious politician also knows that if you state that explicitly, then people will of course object, so instead they enter our minds indirectly by forming the physical environment in which we are living.

MG: As for the architects, can they do their forming in a caring way?
GO: Yes, of course.

MG: How would they, or we, know that the architecture is caring?
GO: I think it is a question of how you legitimate the interference. In the prison, you do so in one way, while in the madhouse, where the point is both to protect people from themselves and to form them in relation to others, you do it in another way. With the caring, it is very much the same. Thus, if you claim that you are building caring architecture you are inevitably legitimating your interference in other people's life. You put yourself in a position where you claim to know what other people need. Not by building a prison to keep them contained but by caring for them, implicitly or explicitly claiming to know more about them from doing whatever we can. These people–those who are in that vulnerable situation–may literally sometimes not even know who they are.

MG: These people would then need a caring architecture that would help them find their way.
GO: Very much in the same way as a small child needs your care. And as a person who is now getting old, I realize that I may soon end up in that situation myself. I am convinced that most of us still want to have our freedoms and our lives. Some of these needs we may not even be aware of, but we certainly don't want to be told what to do. In this caring situation, we want the architecture to be such that we are taken care of without knowing that we are taken care of. We do not want to trip on the threshold, and we would therefore like you to remove it. We would also not like you to put a black carpet in the middle of the room, for too many patients with dementia stepping on a black carpet is like stepping into a black hole. No one would like to be sucked into that abyss.

MG: The architecture, including the interior design, should take care of that.
GO: Yes, and we know this not only from experience but also from current brain research. For example, if we lose our memory we may need help to see the difference between the plate and the porridge. If they are of the same colour, we will not eat the porridge. Many old people are unfortunately senile and some of them are starving to death because they have lost their sense of taste; no wonder that they refuse to eat. Personally, I have long harboured the dream that fifty years from now someone will have invented an aid that will do to the sense of taste what your glasses do to your sight, and my hearing aids do to my bad hearing. Easier said than done, though, partly because the

senses are ordered according to the taboo of not getting too close looking at someone is socially acceptable, licking a stranger is not. One may also note that not too long ago bad hearing was taken as a sign of low intelligence.

MG: It seems that we are now moving from a caring architecture of thresholds, colours and spatial design, towards the human body itself. Certainly, that raises questions about the ethics of a caring architecture.

GO: Well, if we in our caring come too close to people we do so because we have crossed the forbidden line of the taboo. And that is precisely how it should be. Society, in this case operationalized as architecture, has no right to get into me. Yet that is exactly the ethical danger that any caring architecture must face.

MG: Caring architecture raises exo-somatic problems and opportunities in relation to the limits of the human body. How do you conceive of the limits of architecture itself?

GO: The limits of architecture are in the physical structure itself. When the architect designs a building so that I can enter it by a wheelchair, there is an interaction between a physical body and a physical entity. No one can object to that. As long as architecture stays on that level, as long as it tries to adjust physical structures to the caring of the human body, everything is fine.

MG: But that is not only what architecture does.

GO: No, because by designing and constructing physical structures you are deliberately influencing the possibilities for life and behaviour in that building. Once again, this means that architecture operates in the limit between body and mind, material things and social relations. Having norms and regulations for building so that the walls do not fall down is one thing, designing the geography of social interactions is quite another.

MG: And social interaction is what caring architecture designs.

GO: If you do not know where you are, the physical structure should be constructed in such a way that the loss does not matter, that it takes that problem away. Even if you are not able to find your way, you should be respected for who you are, even you may not even know what or where your mouth is. How do you design an environment for that type of situation, not only for the caretakers but for the caregivers as well?

MG: One of several ideological, political and ethical aspects of caring architecture is about who it is designed for, the caretaker or the caregiver?

GO: That is correct, and that raises the problem of who should decide. Obviously, the decisions operate on all levels, but when you have a caring architecture it all comes closer and closer to the individual caretaker. Much of the debate now seems to be more about the caregivers than about the caretakers. The caretakers have relatively little power and it is often their children who feel the need to step in. To have your children take care of you may sometimes be necessary, but it is also a form of caring that is full of deep existential problems.

MG: And both the architecture and the caretaker may appear in many guises.

GO: Yes, and therefore it might be interesting to compare the architecture of care and the architecture of the zoo. Sometimes it seems that there is more concern about the architecture of the zoo than the architecture of the old people´s home. How do you preserve the integrity of these human beings? Indeed, I am occasionally feeling that there is more discussion about the rights of animals than about people who have lost their way. One should of course be very careful here, but there is a point to the point.

MG: Our conversation so far has brought up two crucially important issues.

GO: Yes, the first is about form and process, the relationship between the spatial form and what it does or is intended to do with human processes, the lives that are possible to live in that form. The other issue is an ethical problem that architects rarely confront: architecture is a hidden tool of power. The way you build–even where you place the electric sockets in the room– automatically determines the life that is possible to live in that spatial set-up. You construct a physical structure in order to change people´s minds. Very clear.

MG: So, there is always a politics that comes with and through architecture, in that it promotes human thought-and-action in certain ways. Some may be liberating; some may be confining.

GO: Yes of course, and that is how power always works. Also in architecture, it has a suppressive part and a good part. Power would not be power if it were not contradictory. The danger is that the goodness often gives way to the strictness of the power. For instance, it would be easy to build an escape-proof prison, but no prison-warden ever want to run a jail like that. It would in fact be the worst institution you can have, because what you must not do is to kill the prisoner's wish to escape. Likewise, you must not take away the caretaker´s idea that there is a life outside. To be precise, you must never build so that you kill the faculty of imagination, *the* faculty that makes us human. For example, we do not know what happens in the minds of people with Alzheimer and dementia who by definition have lost their way. Have they also lost their way of imagining another form of life?

MG: In a way, there is the risk that the distance between imagination and the architecture would be reduced almost to zero.

GO: Yes, you might build a caring institution that is so caring that it becomes an escape-proof prison not merely of the body but of the mind as well.

MG: There is then important that caring architecture moves beyond architecture as physical construction.

GO: Yes. If you try to remove the physical foundation of architecture, it becomes more difficult but also much more interesting. Why? Well, because the interest turns precisely towards the relational realm that is located in-between the physical structure and the lives of human beings I have been talking about. Furthermore, one could, by alluding to Immanuel Kant, say that the architecture we know best is the building of the house of pure reason. It follows that we are tempted to use that logic also when we are considering the architecture of caring. And that is wrong.

MG: In other words, thinking architecture in terms of physical structure is not abstract enough?

GO: Of course, not. The way we find our way in the invisible world is by somehow imagining it *as if it were* visible.

MG: To the extent that architecture privileges a reason of physical structures as beings, it would be less well equipped to handle becomings and all the rest that is before or after, or in-between its physical architectonics. It follows that it may benefit from going from nouns to verbs, from architecture to architecturing, much as in the present book care has been turned to caring.

GO: Reflecting from the outside, I imagine that the authors are talking about architecture in that first sense and then expanding into a caring architecture. I do understand and applaud their attempt. However, in that very conception there might at the same time be a temptation to somehow transfer the mode of thought that is in the pure house of reason; since I know how to build a house so it does not tumble down, I too easily conclude that I also know how to build for caring. Humpty Dumpty sat on a wall...

MG: And caring architecture?

GO: Well, a real challenge for caring architecture means that it is not enough to construct a building that does not fall down. The real challenge is instead to build so that the people who are cared for will not fall into the abyss. When the chips are down and the roulette spinning, who is taking it all?

MG: And on whose side is the caring architect when distributing the powers and agencies of caring architecturing?

GO: In my understanding, the architect would be in the infra-thin line of the *Saussurean Bar*. In that conception, caring architecturing is about the glue that at the same time holds us together and keeps us apart, that glue being at the same time both a noun and a verb. On the surface, it is about the physical structure and those who are living within it; deeper down it is about the relations between the architects who have designed the houses and those who are living in them. Once again, we are involved in the dialectics of form and process. In a sense, what I am saying is not merely true, but too true to be true.

MG: True or not, it is a nice way of pausing our conversation.

INTRODUCTION

CATHARINA NORD AND EBBA HÖGSTRÖM

Architecture and institutions

Architecture is hard and inert matter. Walls, roofs, and floors form buildings—by elements composed of solid materials: stone, glass and wood. These elements in turn form rooms, which are quantifiable in metres and square metres, their size defined according to hard, Euclidian spatial concepts, exact to the nearest millimetre. Buildings also have the capacity to restrict and delimit what people *do* within their boundaries; they distribute and direct subjects who, because they see buildings as constituting a self-evident frame for their everyday lives, are unaware of this direction. Thus, despite its apparent hardness, built space is also elusive: its ubiquitous presence and simultaneous absence work to conceal the magnitude and diversity of the influences it exerts over users. Although architecture comprises of tangible and solid matter, the small-scale spatialities this matter produces end up defying their own boundaries and transgressing their own physical content. By virtue of its partnership with those who populate it, whether human or non-human, architecture is therefore both non-tangible and fluid (Yaneva 2012, Dovey 2013, Till 2009).

Institutions constitute perhaps the most difficult of architectures. Their capacity to exert power over, and to forcibly affect, users, reveals their coercive quality as discursive architectural models and practices: institutional architecture in this sense can restrict ways of thinking and acting and privilege certain options over others (cf. Foucault 1977, Goffman 1961). Institutions are often "big things", both in the sense of being massive buildings in themselves and in their (international) proliferation as design models (Jacobs 2006). Hospitals, asylums, correctional facilities, national and political institutions and urban megaprojects are all ascribed particular capacities to impress, punish and govern citizens, and perhaps to care for their inmates (Dovey 2008, Markus 1993, Vale 2014). Although, it is sometimes difficult to link this caring and empathetic attitude to the austerity and rigidity of the architectural space of such institutions (Markus 1993, Åman 1976, Godfrey 1955).

It would of course be a serious mistake to assess the institutions of another time in accordance with the humanist values of the present. However, if older architectural models survive in the design of contemporary hospitals, facilities for the care of the aged, in psychiatric facilities, etc., can we then presume that the thoughts and practices that led to their production also survived in one way or another, by being embedded in architectural space? John Law argues that thought and matter—and architectural space constitutes both—are deeply entwined. He writes, "It is the generation of material effects that lies at the heart of the modernist project of self-reflexivity" (Law 1994, 139). Taking into account such effects, this book aims to open up new pathways for thinking about and discussing *institutional architectural space*. Borrowing from Law (1994), one point of departure for this work lies in our understanding of institutions as being iterated by the performance of matter, space, ideas and people through certain modes of "ordering". Institutions and architecture are here seen as intimately intertwined in a manner that in fact bypasses the architectural object. This standpoint challenges a view, which positions the institution as a representation, a repeated model of architectural design and of certain discursive rationalities. Instead, we choose to address institutions as *performances*, to consider what they *do* rather than what they *mean* (Dovey 2013, Jacobs and Merriman 2011).

The architecture of institutions has changed dramatically in the last 50 years. The austere, impressive and strict institutional architecture of yesteryear has now been abandoned, giving way to other design models. The so-called "healing architecture" of newly designed hospitals endows spaces such as the lobby with a welcoming atmosphere, and places aesthetic emphasis on patient rooms where family members may even be able to stay overnight (Wagenaar 2006). Homes for the elderly have turned into assisted living facilities, in which older people no longer share their rooms with strangers and can socialise with fellow residents in ambitiously designed public areas with high-quality interior furnishings (Regnier 2002). Even the architecture of the most "hardcore" of all institutions—the prison—has been transformed in order to manifest humanist ideals such as respect for the individual and the humane treatment of inmates (Chantraine 2010, Fairweather and McConville 2000). Despite these shifts, changes in institutional architecture are far more complex than what is suggested at first glance. Far from a simple replacement of the old with the new, architectural design approaches are intertwined in intricate and often contradictory ways (Street 2012). The changes witnessed in institutional architectural design may in this sense be less profound than they seem, and in fact may simply reflect the greater influence exerted by culture rather than of any fundamental alteration in the way that we think about medical spaces. Thus, we encounter a situation wherein new hospital designs may on the one hand reclaim medical and organisational ideas from the early 20th century, whilst at the same time integrating commercial environments in their structures (Adams 2007). The latter spaces (shopping malls, etc.) are often to some extent cut off from the rest of the hospital, with the primary aim of securing a patient base rather than making any real difference in relation to the wellbeing of the sickest and weakest (Sloane 1994). Like the healing architecture of the hospital, the "humane prison" can also be questioned with respect to contemporary societal needs for security and the consequent incarceration of "dangerous" inmates (Chantraine 2010). Similarly, the redesign of psychiatric hospitals, which have for several decades been the target for changes in size, location, timeframes and levels of control under labels such as *de-*, *trans-* and *re*institutionalisation (Parr 2008, Högström 2012), must also be considered as a complex layering rather than a replacement of old with new. The policy of deinstitutionalising mental healthcare has played out very different in different contexts, and has resulted in more or less successful community-based alternatives to asylum-based care, and this constitutes a further complexity, which must be taken into account (Gleeson and Kearns 2001).

Despite ambitions to create a new institutional architecture, the examples addressed in the chapters of this book—namely, a hospital (Björgvinsson and Sandin), a residential care home for teenagers (Severinsson), and assisted living (Nord, Andersson) and mental health facilities (Ross, McGeachan, Högström)—reinforce the on-going importance of older commitments to "reform" those admitted into institutional care. Thus, despite the isolation imposed on the individuals admitted into their care, the primary aim of such institutions is still to restore wellbeing, improve conduct and in most cases, rehabilitate individuals into the community of the healthy and the "normal". It is argued that the modern project was imbued by a preoccupation with the establishment of social order, embedded for instance in social engineering, with the aim of handling the ambiguous and the deviant (Bauman 1991). Traditionally, institutions were assigned the role in this context of "collecting and confining those who in one way or another could introduce chaos into the social order" (Markus 1993, 95). The chapters of this book reinforce the importance of this inheritance, describing facilities in which this commitment is still discernible, where "awkward" and sick people spend time severed from the community in order to become healthy and well-functioning citizens. Whilst the older institutional role of keeping up a given social order is therefore possible to trace in contemporary projects, the scholarly preoccupation with order has largely been eclipsed by an interest in the relationship between power and resistance in institutions, often building on the theoretical work of Michel Foucault (Dovey 2008, Allen 2003, Sharp et al. 2000). Power thus appears in this anthology in its oppressive form but also in more obscure and opaque versions, as "manipulation" or even "seduction". Whilst acknowledging the importance of previous literature, we are not here primarily interested in tracing the social order as a product of the societal endeavour of institutions; rather, as we hinted at earlier, we adopt a view of space as an act of "ordering" as advocated by Law (1994) and by Hetherington (1997). As such, we contend—with Jacobs and Merriman (2011, 212, emphasis in orginal)—that "social order [i]s an outcome not of impervious, omnipotent, *out there* structures or systems, but *right here* coordinated (although not always rational) agreements and arrangements based in contingently formed skills and interpretations". Our interest takes us "right here", inside the walls of our institutions, with a focus on the everyday practices performed by architectural space and other matter in cooperation with the people who live and work in institutions for shorter or longer periods. Our aim is to elucidate how architectural space in institutions is involved in processes of complex ordering—the kind of ordering which destabilises order, as it were—thereby hopefully contributing a more detailed and nuanced image of what it is that is happening in institutional care today.

In this task, we also wish to emphasise the political implications of both institutions and of the concept of care. How a society treats their members in need of care—be they physically or mentally ill, old and frail, or young and deviant—mirrors the values of that society. Lawson (2007, 5) points out that the marginalisation of care in a time of individualism is a political act, which supports "the myth that our successes are achieved as autonomous individuals". In light of these comments, the criticism of institutions, which emerged in the 1960s and 1970s in line with discourses of "autonomy" in fact, appears to have largely constituted an act of stereotyping which has labelled the institution as being, above all, repressive (cf. Gleeson and Kearns 2001). Even if being "an autonomous individual" involved the recognition of justice and universal rights, care institutions were not seen to support such values under such a critique. To go "right here", inside the institutional walls, should be read as a desire to challenge these now out-dated stereotypes and to advance a more complex, multifaceted understanding of institutions as spatial, organisational, affective and political configurations where care, cure, control, agency, power, hopes and possibilities all merge.

Architectural geography and non-representational theory

This book sets out to show how people and spaces are able to negotiate, and often to challenge, the norms and patterns embedded in the intersection of architecture and institutions. A non-representational perspective allows the emergent, flexible and mouldable practices in which institutional architecture is defied, contested and transformed to be brought into view (Anderson and Harrison 2010a, Thrift 2008). The label *non-representational theory* loosely gathers together theorists who stress relations and the contingent and emergent dimensions of the world (eg. DeLanda 2006, Latour 2005, Deleuze and Guattari 2004, Dewsbury et al. 2002, Barad 2007). In transforming the noun 'being' to the verb 'becoming' this set of theories make way within human geography and architectural research for concepts such as the *spacing* and the *practising* of architecture (Beyes and Steyaert 2011, Jacobs and Merriman 2011). Space as spacing "entails a move from representational strategies of extracting representations of the world to embodied apprehensions of the everyday performing of space, to different enactments of ... geographies" (Beyes and Steyaert 2011, 47). Whilst we acknowledge that spaces are produced in the flow of everyday social life (Lefebvre 1991), we advocate that they must also be seen as being in themselves capable of production (Jacobs 2006). In developing these spatial concerns, non-representational theorists emphasise the distributed nature of agency, rejecting views which position human experience at the self-evident centre of all occurrences, ascribing agentic capacities instead to a far broader field which includes (dead) material, artefacts and even space itself (Wylie 2010, Bennett 2009). In this book, we aim to look beyond architecture and buildings as mere objects, and instead apply a relational spatial perspective, which positions architectural space as an actor and co-producer. Buildings, we argue, have agentic properties in that they do things to and with people. In this task, we sympathise with Jacobs and Merriman (2011, 211-212) wish to "animate architecture such that it is understood not simply as an accomplishment (or artefact) of human doing, but as an on-going process of holding together and, inevitably or even coincidentally, not holding together". Architecture is held together by practices embedded in space, and the chapters in this book address the many guises in which care practices are made manifest in and through architectural space. This "holding" is illustrated in situations wherein older institutions or architectural spaces that were originally built for another (completely different) function are literally held together by the introduction of new caring purposes. Taking inspiration from an architectural geography that profits a non-representational theoretical perspective, the studies of diverse institutional architectures and their holding capacities that are brought together in this book are, we believe, capable of "taking on board a conceptual awareness of the material, embodied, affective and minor configurations of space" (Beyes and Steyaert 2011, 56).

Inhabiting, designing, mattering and knowing—all notions raised by Jacobs and Merriman (2011)—constitute themes that appear and reappear throughout the book, in chapters which demonstrate (sometimes subtly and sometimes emphatically) the entwined, inseparable and co-constitutive relation of these processes in relation to one another. *Inhabiting* is an everyday practice; "[b]uildings inhabit our lives just as we inhabit them" (Jacobs and Merriman 2011, 214), and inhabitation occurs in the minor events and situations through which institutional care evolves, revolves and rebels. Notions of inhabitation are present in all the chapters of the book and this constitutes a key concept for the anthology as a whole. *Designing*—in terms of both the act itself, as well as the significance of representations in design and even the potential marginalisation of design ideas—also emerges as a recurring theme, with several chapters addressing designing as a major force in shaping the everyday, even to the point of overt manipulation. When it comes to notions of *Mattering,* both senses of the word resonate within the book. Matter (that is, the hard material stuff, the objects and the architectural elements) *matters* to what emerges from the "intra-actions" that produce institutional care (cf. Barad 2003). Closely connected to matters of concern are affects, emotions, values and attachments, which come about through the employment of tangible stuff in practice (Jacobs and Merriman 2011, 217). Finally, objects and physical spaces are also depicted here as mouldable shapeshifters, engaged in dynamic performances, which include numerous discursive positions. We adopt a pragmatic approach in relation to the concept of *Knowing*, which emerges through the work in this book as predominantly constituting a practice that is negotiated and developed in spatial performances and sometimes in utterances made by people. Jacobs and Merriman (2011, 219) emphasise the disciplinary differences between geographers and architects in matters relating to knowing, and building on that discussion, we seek to draw architecture and geography more closely together, since "buildings are a fundamental geographical setting" (Kraftl 2010, 403). Our aim includes participating in the research dialogue that Jacobs and Merriman wish to see between these two disciplines, thereby adding to knowledge about both and about the scientific crossroads where they meet, interact and entwine.

Caring architecture

A number of scholars have linked caring and therapeutic effects to space and architecture with the support of terms such as *geographies of care, landscapes of care* and *therapeutic landscapes* (Milligan and Wiles 2010, Conradson 2005, 2003, McCormack 2003). These concepts encompass a wide range of caring spaces at scales that extend from the global to the local and that must be seen in the broader context of their political and ideological ambitions, their proliferation and distribution across private and public sectors, the form of care and the carers they support, and their ability to produce and reproduce gendered and (un)equal patterns of care. This research highlights the affective, emotional, material and spatial aspects of receiving and giving care (Milligan and Wiles 2010). Without entering an in-depth discussion of these particular concepts, we want to unearth the underlying premise presented by these scholars: that it is necessary to look at the complexity of caring situations; to take into account the relational aspects of care; and to see architectural space as an event, as something coming into being (Dewsbury 2000).

"[A]rchitecture is always a partial project, an unfinished project, by definition incomplete … You could even say that architecture is always a failure; it never accomplishes what it intends" (Lash et al. 2009, 10). Much of the literature addressing architecture for institutional care has normative connotations and is presented as recommendations, descriptions of best practice or guidelines (eg. Regnier 2002, Fairweather and McConville 2000, Wagenaar 2006). This approach to the architectural design of institutions, in which quality is often defined as a stable category ascribing certain values to both space and care, implies that a building is finished when it is completed, the point at which all endeavours are "accomplished". Such assumptions attempt to catch and imprison properties and situations that can neither be confined nor immobilised in this way. By applying a non-representational approach to care and architecture such as the one advocated through this book, we arrive at a different understanding of these captured moments, seeing them rather as parts of an on-going performance. Care is work that is repeated and tested many times until it reaches an acceptable quality. As such, it is *tinkering*, an unfinished practice involving the carer's affective, empathetic and improvising capacities in which good and bad become part of a continuous process (Mol, Moser, and Pols 2010). Caring qualities and architectural space are produced simultaneously, in the very moment in which care is carried out (Nord 2015). A further normative belief that must be dealt with is that of *person-centred care*, which the benchmark in debate surrounding care today is. The proponents of person-centred care stress that the individual patient's needs and wishes should be the leading determination and ethical core in every caring encounter (McCormack and McCance 2011). We argue that when this encounter is entwined in the contingency of place, matter and people, the category of absolute patient focus will be destabilised by unforeseen forces and incidents in the caring event. How then does person-centred care appear in the context of spatio-material processes? Is person-centred care a relevant notion at all? To come to terms with such moral issues, we here focus on a form of care practice based on a "pre-personally emergent, but personally implicated affective space of ethical sensibility", which "shifts the burden of the ethical away from the effort to do justice to individual subjects, and towards a commitment to develop a *fidelity to the event*" (McCormack 2003, 496, 502 referring to Badiou 2002, italics in original). This does not rule out a person-centred care approach, but gives it an entirely new meaning by embracing the totality of the caring event. We contend, with McCormack (2003, 502), that "[t]his is in no way an anti-human position". Rather, it opens up the possibility that the individual body is something more than just that body involved in care-receiving, but rather enmeshed in emergent relations of caring "as that through which new spaces of thinking and moving may come into being" (502 referring to Dewsbury 2000).

The non-representational approach to care can contribute to destabilising the normative polarity in assessments of institutional quality and of ethical judgement. The comparison between institutional care and community-based care has often been framed in terms of a false opposition of "good" and "bad" (Gleeson and Kearns 2001), echoing the normative ethical standards on which this dichotomy is pinned. The chapters in this book aim to discuss the complexity and inconsistencies present in institutions, casting doubt on moral certitude and on the issue of what high quality architectural space is. Architecture is always incomplete (Lash et al. 2009, 10). It is this incompleteness that embodies architectural agency and allows it to act and to "'act otherwise' or lead to other possible futures" (Doucet and Cupers 2009, 1): either next minute, tomorrow or years into the future. Our hope is that the perspectives of non-representational theory will reveal institutional architecture and care "acting otherwise", providing pertinent examples of situations in which relational and transformative conditions emerge (or fail to emerge) as *caring architecture*.

Contributions

We hope this book will reveal a new dimension within the established topic of institutional architecture and institutional care. The themes explored within the different contributions interlink and overlap in a manner that illustrates the complex, diverse and sometimes even contradictory views possible in relation to institutional architecture and institutional care. Despite their differences, though, the contributions are united by a shared conception of architecture as a process of spacing rather than as an immobile object.

The anthology provides a series of examples of specific care features in relation to a series of specific architectural forms. The authors of the chapters—who come from the fields of architecture, design, geography and social work—together demonstrate the variety of ways in which care practices and care discourses make use of architecture and other materials in order to change and fluctuate, to stabilise and to capture new meanings by negotiations that take place in and with space. Each of the chapters highlights in a different manner how locations, buildings, rooms, regulations, policies or even organisational structures frame the way in which care is provided and how the experience of receiving care is perceived and performed. Readers will thus encounter not only a vast range of specific examples but also a multiplicity of theoretical perspectives, which reflect the range of positions that have given birth to non-representational theory itself (Thrift 2008). The work of important theorists like Henri Lefebvre, Gilles Deleuze and Felix Guattari, Bruno Latour and Michel Callon, and Karen Barad are thus repeatedly cited. In this way, we invite dialogue with a number of key scholars in this field.

In the first chapter, Erling Björgvinsson and Gunnar Sandin deal with hospitalised patients who are faced with a brutal reorientation of their normal spatial needs and preferences and are forced to adjust spatially to a new environment. The patients, Björgvinsson and Sandin reveal, soon start to rearrange their own spatial situation according to their personal needs and the site-specific circumstances, in ways which not only include replacing the institutional objects at hand with their private possessions, but also adjusting to the presence and needs of the staff and other patients. This chapter discusses the type of spatial manoeuvring and the norms that emerge when the patients negotiate and align with a hospital's culture.

In Chapter 2, Susanne Severinsson provides a *diffractive reading* of an art studio in order to examine the fluctuating and stabilising aspects of room and materiality in residential care for troubled young people. She explores, through various discursive lenses, what kinds of knowledge and subjectivities are produced in the art studio when they are looked upon as networks and translations of actants: as discourses, humans and materialities. The focus is on what is constituted or performed in emergent relations between teenagers, teachers, objects and material space captures both the stabilising social effects of materiality as well as its complexity and flow.

In Chapter 3, Catharina Nord explores three essential goals of caring—autonomy, privacy and dignity—by taking a closer looking at the historical, architectural roots of assisted living with the support of the Deleuzian/Guattarian concept *stratum*. Care is conceptualised in this chapter as *tinkering*, a practice that develops with the situation and that is largely an improvisation in order to find the best way of doing things. This way of understanding care reveals the work done between set routines, opening the door to redefining the quality of care which emerges from an assemblage of diverse materials and actors, including architectural space.

Chapters 4 and 5 deal with the design of historical asylum space. In the fourth chapter, Kim Ross writes about the engineering of *affective atmospheres* within the interior of Scotland's 19th-century asylum spaces. With the aim of both controlling and curing, this act of planning and designing spaces to exert architectural influence over the asylum population was a highly politicised move by those in positions of authority. The moral, medical and hygienic dimensions of the discourse ultimately outline its institutional geography, and the profound influence it had on asylum layout and design, with the internal (and external) spaces of the asylum being engineered to affect the behaviour of the patients. Ross also brings to the fore the difficulties of using a non-representational theoretical perspective within historical research, suggesting a conceptual approach by looking at spaces as being *potentially* affective.

In the fifth chapter, Cheryl McGeachan acquaints us with the work of the Scottish psychiatrist Ronald David Laing who became internationally renowned for his work on humanist approaches to psychiatric care. Laing developed a strong reliance on the healing properties of asylum space and this chapter to reveals the differing ways in which Laing (re)configures psychiatric and therapeutic spaces through investigating *the Rumpus Room* experiment. McGeachan's specifically turns her attention to the complex interconnections between the spaces of care, the psychiatric encounter and the worlds of individuals experiencing mental ill(health) in which new subjectivities emerge.

Chapter 6 constitutes a discussion about the usability of architectural space in a changing and dynamic environment, specifically within the case of assisted living. Morgan Andersson presents *usability* as the result of normative design processes and the daily use of restricted common spaces for weak and elderly individuals. He argues that despite spatial limitations, the facility's usability is created in continual negotiations between the environment and users in the performance of spaces, artefacts and residents. Henri Lefebvre's three aspects of space are here used as a conceptual frame for discussing the tensions between conceived, perceived and lived space.

In the seventh chapter seven, Ebba Högström looks into the   difficulties of   translating   specific   spatial   experiences   into   general   design recommendations. The chapter revolves around organisation, design, experiences and representations of the *Saltsjöbaden Mental Health Centre (SMHC)*, which opened in 1975 as part of the decentralisation movement in Sweden. The design of the centre's premises was anchored in a discourse of openness, equality and accessibility. However, the premises soon became a contested space, open to negotiation and conflicting rationalities. Consequently, when SMHC was used in guidelines for the "new psychiatry" by *SPRI*, a national institute for planning and rationalising health care, most of its relational potentialities were occluded.

With a little help from our colleagues

The book also includes commentary texts from experienced theorists from three relevant disciplinary fields, human geography, caring sciences and architecture. Gunnar Olsson and Martin Gren set out to contend the whole idea of caring architecture by their dialogue about the formative qualities on peoples' behaviour and thinking of physical structures by which goodness and powers become blurred in dubious alliances. Chris Philo continues this theme by presenting the historical context of institutional care where no doubt coercion has been a central aspect. However, he also discusses the efforts from within the field itself to come to terms with inhuman ways of treating vulnerable patients by developing new spaces and caring practices. Ingunn Moser presents the relational embeddedness of care in material and spatial circumstances from which qualities, subjects and agencies arise. She also argues for stronger links between Science and Technology Studies and architecture that could form new fruitful constellations, ideas and issues. Albena Yaneva follows this line of thought by showing how the agentic qualities of architecture emerge from the contexts in which it is embedded. She concludes the book with a plea for a careful attention to architecture to enable it to care. We need to care for architecture.

COMMENTARY II

COVERTLY ENTANGLED LINES

CHRIS PHILO

Into the institutional field

Pimbo's other exciting discovery was that of patients' behaviour in the new barber-shop. The shop, complete with strip lighting, chromium-plated hair rinsing equipment, shining new basins, large friendly mirrors, had taken the place of ward shaving and hair trim. A nice upholstered leather chair afforded new comfort, but it was the transformation which took place as the old demented man would take his seat. It seemed to Pimbo that the years had been rolled back. The patient would assume a new dignity, head held back, he would push out his cheek at the appropriate time to coincide with the razor. During the haircutting, heads would be turned obligingly when so required, and in general everything was done to assist the barber. (Unwin 1976, 32)

This passage comes from a "novel"–essentially a memoir–recounting the experiences of Pimbo, the nickname for Jack Freestone, himself evidently the stand-in for book's author, F.T. Unwin, from his days as a student psychiatric nurse in a British mental hospital of the late-1950s/early-1960s (Fig. CII:1). The passage encapsulates certain connections between material space and forms of care, arguably speaking directly to a theme of *caring architectures*, if here in the very specific circumstances of (re)designing a mental hospital "barber shop" for cutting the hair of male patients. More narrowly, what is intimated is a highly embodied instance in creating the "spatial politics of affect" (Thrift 2004), in that here ostensibly small alterations to the material spaces of the institution–a newly-fitted out "barber shop", with accoutrements akin to those of a modern barber shop on an everyday high street–foster an *affective atmosphere* (Anderson 2009) which tangibly infuses how the patients comport themselves. Heads held back and cheeks puffed out, as if with a rediscovery of some lost sense of pride in self and appearance, the patients "assume[d] a new dignity". Rather than the perfunctory shave-and-trim on the ward, the barest of caring acts merely enacting hygienic control over the resident population, the patients were now allowed to visit this new site in the hospital, momentarily becoming something different, cared for humanly, even aesthetically, and with time taken on them as *more-than-just* patients. Similar results were reported for the equivalent "female shop", offering "[w]ash and set, perms and styling," and Pimbo "reckoned that a touch of the outside world had kindled the flame which once flickered before hospitalisation" (Unwin 1976, 32).

Unwin's recollections are of an intriguing period in post-WWII mental health reform, entailing dramatic shifts in the institutional geography of mental health care, as the earlier *asylum* system–dependent on set-apart institutions, massive built structures usually sited in splendid rustic isolation– was gradually being dismantled on the way to the more familiar *post-asylum* system of today (in most Western countries)–operated through overlapping networks of services and facilities, dispersed, sometimes fragmented, normally couched as *community*-based and *community*-facing (eg. Wolch and Philo 2000, Högström 2012, Parr 2008). For Pimbo, though, the old asylum-hospital remained his primary site of work and encounter for what he termed, intriguingly, his "being in the field" (Unwin 1976, 125): a "field" where he learned his trade from the spaces, patients and staff, and where he acquired, as per the title of his book, "dew on [his] feet" (145). Indeed, the book's events were set primarily within the orbit of Fulbourn Hospital, once the Cambridgeshire County Lunatic Asylum (opened in the 1860s), located a few miles into the countryside outside of Cambridge, premier city of British learning, and originally sealed in behind "forbidding walls"–albeit "the high stone wall which once surrounded the entire hospital [was] now long since a thing of the past" (7). As this remark suggests, however, the spaces of the old asylum-hospital were changing before Pimbo's eyes: the external walls had come down, as too the walls around the old exercise yard which had once "provid[ed] violent patients just enough space in which to burn their aggression" (18), and the doors had been unlocked ("'There are no locked doors now–it's observation that counts'": (8), quoting Tim, an experienced nurse). Indeed, "[t]hings were rapidly changing in the hospital, and Pimbo was seeing fresh faces walking casually around the grounds and corridors, faces that a few years ago were staring from top room windows, as though characters from a Victorian novel" (142). He particularly noted new ways in which patients started to inhabit the institution: "once never allowed to leave their wards", suddenly there they were "in the corridors" with a purpose, perhaps heading to and from the canteen to purchase food and drinks, no longer "mak[ing] a dash through a half-open door" but "walk[ing] contentedly along brightly painted corridors" (59-60). This was no longer a solely carceral establishment, a spatiality of enclosure (Jeffrey, McFarlane, and Vasudevan 2012) predicated on fixing patients within surveilled bounds from which they could never stray alone, but rather one providing a limited "geography of licence" (Goffman 1961) and permitting a small measure of independent movement, encounter and choice.

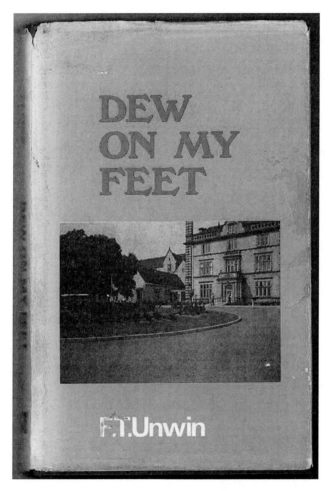

Fig. Cll:1. Jacket cover of *Dew on my Feet.* Reprinted by permission from Arthur H Stockwell Ltd.

Traces of the original asylum were disappearing–"[o]ld wards, once lively, housing violent and personality disorders, had been phased out" (Unwin 1976, 142)–and new spaces, more varied and in some cases loosely reminiscent of more "normal" places of being and doing, were appearing in their stead. Long-stay patients were discouraged, and more attention focussed on "acute admissions", as in Kent House, which was deliberately lent a more home-like quality supposed to avoid the resonances of the older prison-asylum:

> Kent House in itself certainly looked an inviting place, rather in the lines of a hotel. Beautiful drapes, coffee tables in liberal supply, television, and a lounge furnished with settees and chairs all of which were top class furnishings. ... An excellent dining-room, separate tables, with choice of menu, piped music, and again with furniture of top class. (90)

Spatial arrangements, including décor and furnishings, all played their part in creating what, once again, might be deemed an affective atmosphere, definitely engineered, not mere happenstance. Another new space was the Deighton Centre, "a large unit dealing with occupational therapy for inmates and day patients" (106), where the most capable patients would undertake useful work "such as packing sterile dressings, stripping plastic rawlplugs from their embryonic state, into a useable neatly packed commodity ready for consumer use" (108). Pimbo reckoned this space–he called it the Fulbourn residents' "new found haven"–to offer "a great change from the olden days where lines of apathetic patients sat passively between meals," now replaced by "an atmosphere reeking of honest endeavour" (107). Moreover:

> [t]he therapeutic value of this did wonders in rejuvenating worn limbs, stroke-ridden muscles, and giving gnarled fingers a new lease of life. Patients were stirred from chair-bound senility into a world of strip-lighting, coloured plugs, bingo, sing-songs, coach outings, and renewed acquaintances with old friends and neighbours. (107)

While there are elements here, in retrospect, that might strike as among the more unappealing aspects of an artificially collectivised "hospital life", they nonetheless speak clearly of attempts–I would call them genuine attempts, even while wishing to retain a critical edge (see below)–at enlisting all manner of spatial tactics, to do with form and affordances, in creating meaningful existence and maybe even rehabilitation leading to "cure" and "release".

Finally, alongside the breaking up of the original big blocky asylum spaces–into smaller, more diverse "houses", wards and units, together with spaces like canteens and barber shops–there was also some dispersion of the institution away from its site on the Fulbourn estate. As the walls came down and day patients were allowed in, so the first faltering steps were being taken with *care in the community* initiatives. Recognising that some patients "should be capable of living outside the hospital," so "little houses had been started in which the better type of patients might live together under casual supervision" (111). More fully, Pimbo described this first stage in what was to become the hegemonic deinstitutionalisation movement in Western mental health care from the 1950s/1960s to the present day:

> Little houses within a short distance of the hospital had been opened as starting points for patients, whose eventual discharge was well in the offing. Living together, under limited supervision, the patients cooked, shopped, and managed to be almost self-contained. Patients working outside the hospital, to return at night[,] had long since been under way. (142)

This was deinstitutionalisation in a distinctly minor key, of course, orchestrated from *within* the institution and retaining a host of older institutional motifs, including ongoing "supervision" and "observation", as in the quote from Tim, the old nurse, but it would be mistaken not to detect here all manner of seeds that would later flower into the multiple spaces of *post-asylum geographies* (themselves of course not without their own many limitations).

Finding Unwin's book held a particular resonance for me personally. While an undergraduate student at Cambridge in the early-1980s, I was part of student volunteer groups who visited the Fulbourn Hospital to provide "normal" contacts and distractions, mainly for short-term residents of a young person's unit, sometimes taking them on trips into the city, to go punting, even to the pub. Pimbo even recalls contributions made by "voluntary groups of students from the colleges of near-by Cambridge" (31). The book has long languished on my book-shelves awaiting a moment to be more critically consulted, however, but precisely that moment has arrived with the invitation to draft a scene-setting chapter to this fascinating volume on the entanglements of care, control and other dynamics in the institutional architectural space of hospitals, asylums, homes for the infirm elderly, units for the disturbed young and many others in the same broad institutional family. What Pimbo recounts in detail are early efforts at crafting a modern "healing architecture" predicated on a spectrum from grand manipulations of geometry ("opening closed spaces", Wolpert 1976) through to tiny tinkerings with shapes, decorations and furnishings. Many such efforts–great and small; system-wide or local; self-consciously experimental or more happenstance– are explored in the current volume, and at the same time many broad-brush themes of both wide societal relevance or with serious critical-academic import are being tackled. In my own scene-setting here, I will try to weave in some comments on the specific chapters in this volume, as in the paragraph immediately below, as well as looking to frame some of the broader themes that, for me, most tellingly ripple throughout the pages that follow.

While the Fulbourn experience recounted here anticipates later developments, it also echoes earlier interventions in asylum-based *moral treatment* and its architectural-locational dimensions from at least the later-eighteenth century (Philo 2004, esp. Chapt. 6; see also below). Thus, there are links to what Kim Ross, in her chapter (Chapt. 4), compellingly identifies as the purposeful engineering of affective atmospheres in the Scottish district asylums from the 1860s onwards, a form of spatial engineering that so clearly anticipates, in so many ways, the practices of post-WWII asylum reform. There is arguably nothing in Pimbo's account as dramatic as what is narrated in Cheryl McGeachan's chapter (Chapt. 5) when she tackles R.D. Laing's celebrated, if contested, experiment with the so-called *rumpus room* at Gartnavel Hospital (originally the Glasgow Royal Asylum) during the mid-1950s, although it is perhaps not such a stretch from the rumpus room to an emphasis on unlocked wards, opportunities for patients to come and go almost as they pleased around the hospital's many spaces, and constant attempts to inculcate relatively "normal" forms of spatialised sociability: "Pimbo felt that the true nature of the patient was shown" when routinely engaging with "that which resembled most a normal way of living; eating, sleeping, arguing and enjoying another's company" (Unwin 1976, 132). Similarly, there is nothing here that directly aligns with what Ebba Högström's chapter (Chapt. 7) addresses, the Saltsjöbaden Mental Health Centre (SMHC) in Nacka municipality, open near Stockholm in the mid-to late-1970s, with its suite of experimental spaces designed to allow flexibility of use, subversion of hierarchies and the enactment of "potentials, contestations and differentiations". Yet, even in the Fulbourn case as retold by Pimbo, there are hints at spaces which were not *always* to be about calm, rational order, keeping a "lid" on people and situations, but could involve some of the challenge and unpredictability of the SMHC: "A few nurses believed that[,] given a proper setting where perhaps an aspect of histrionics prevailed, a delusion could be broken" (Unwin 1976, 87); while Pimbo also related instances where patients and spaces might be allowed to remain wonderfully "other", as in the case of Charlie, an ex-furniture remover, who "would spend most of his time pointing at beds and furniture, moving them willy-nilly to all corners of the city, in a fantasy of pre-hospital memories" (39 [with echoes of the dazzling claims made by Laws (2012) about "mad work"]).

Additionally, the Fulbourn story, notably in the description of the Deighton Centre, gestures to the creation of those (now unloved, even unwanted) communal spaces that are the focus of the chapters on assisted living accommodation (care homes) for elderly people by, respectively, Catharina Nord (Chapt. 3) and Morgan Andersson (Chapt. 6). It even dovetails with the attention lent by Susanne Severinsson (Chapt. 2) to the spaces of possibility–ones resisting over-direction of activity or over-interpretation of actions–within a residential care home for troubled teenagers: indeed, Pimbo was invited to consider working in "a new adolescent unit" where "keys, ... restrictive measures are on the way out" (Unwin 1976, 143), where "sensitivity groups" would permit unstructured, non-moralistic discussions on all manner of personal issues, and where the nurse "will gain respect and ability to help from a less detached distance" (145).

Care and control, again

> Emphasis on the long-term history of the rise of confinement precludes any sort of explanation *only* in terms of benevolence *or* the wish to control. In reality both may have existed simultaneously, with varying ratios in different periods. ... On the one hand, repression as such always implies attempts to control the population. On the other hand, the ways of repression changed considerably and these changes, whatever else they meant, also reflected a transformation of sensibilities. A closer understanding of these inter-dependencies could contribute to our understanding of the long-term processes involved, which continue into the present. (Spierenburg 1984, 7)

This claim comes from Pieter Spierenburg's introduction to his intriguing 1984 edited collection on "the emergence of carceral institutions", specifically European "prisons, galleys and lunatic asylums", between 1500 and 1900. Spierenburg presents the task of the collection as "a mapping based on data from archival research" (6), but also as one permeated by a critical-interpretative move designed to overcome a simplistic dichotomy between either naïve progressivism (convinced of ever-increasing humanitarianism in the institutional realm) or its reverse (convinced of its ongoing, possibly deepening, repressive tendencies). Instead of "humanitarian benevolence", the latter emphasises "a gloomy modern technique of total control" (6):

> The resulting opposition between the idiom of reform and the idiom of control is actually an opposition between good and bad. The issue is that of the nobleness versus the wickedness of prison-builders, administrators, lawyers and legislators. This dichotomy is regrettable and should be overcome. (6)

Hence the first quotation borrowed above from Spierenburg, suggesting the need to detect the balance–the "varying ratios in different periods" and, I might add, places–between a basket of what might be termed more benevolent gestures (care, reform, compassion) and another full of more authoritarian demands (control, discipline, dispassion). More complexly, he proposes that these two baskets "may have existed simultaneously" in many institutions to the point of being inter-dependent, the one, care, integrally bound into the accomplishment of the other, control, and *vice versa*. To speak of care and control as entirely different processes is thus in error: rather, each folds into its other, perhaps not in every case but in very many, engendering institutional spaces conditioned precisely by this deep doubling of care-and-control logics.

As is now familiar, histories written of prisons, asylums, poorhouses and related facilities have often tended towards a progressivist recounting, identifying an increasingly benign, humane and indeed "caring" set of ideas and practices coursing through, and shaping, the institutional spaces in question. Three examples from among many on my bookshelves can be referenced: in a collection of local history essays on social welfare in the English county of Hertfordshire, Steven King's introductory essay concludes "that Hertfordshire really was a caring county" (King 2013, 11); opening her remembering of Storthes Hall Hospital, originally the fourth West Riding of Yorkshire (England) public county lunatic asylum (opened in 1904), Anne Linwood remarks how "I have been constantly reminded of the fact that, whatever care was given, it was believed to be the best at that time and should be seen in context" (Linwood 2003, 5); while in the epilogue to his history of Claybury Hospital, originally the fourth Middlesex (England) public county lunatic asylum (opened in 1893), subtitled a "a century of caring", Eric Pryor celebrates "the splendid work and dedication of the early pioneers who preceded us, for without their heroic efforts to establish and improve the service, the care of today's mentally ill would be immeasurably the poorer" (Pryor 1993, 168). Both Linwood and Pryor had been on the mental health nursing staff of their respective institutions, in which regard they overlap intriguingly with Unwin's "story" of Pimbo at Fulbourn Hospital. Such local and "in-house" histories, often authored by individuals closely associated with the facilities under study, can too easily be dismissed by the professional historian with his or her avowedly more critical eye, but in practice such histories–with their deep concern for detail, including spatial-environmental detail (maps, plans and illustrations of buildings and grounds pepper the three books just mentioned)–frequently provide an extremely nuanced, if not theorised, picture of how care, control and spaces actually and always co-mingled "on the ground". Consider the opening quote above from Pimbo (Unwin), for instance, where the caring aspects of the new hairdressing space, returning bodily pride to the long-institutionalised, were nonetheless *also* in step with enhancing control over these patients during what could otherwise be uneasy, confrontational moments on the ward: as Pimbo recalls, "heads would be turned obligingly ... and in general everything was done to assist the barber." In this minute observation, care and control are indeed totally intertwined, the one shading seamlessly into the other, an acute consciousness of which was probably lost on Pimbo (Unwin) but is arguably of huge relevance to the historian or historical geographer of *madness* and its treatment.

This small instance can be cast in the much broader orbit of inquiries by those more critical or radical scholars of social welfare setting themselves against the progressivist perspective in the field. More precisely, I would situate it in the horizon of Michel Foucault's dramatic intervention in studying the history of madness, which, as is now well-known, essentially turned the progressivist account on its head by proposing instead a regressivist account, wherein the plight of those positioned as *mad* or "unreasonable" becomes– over the *longue durée* of European philosophical-cultural change from the 1600s onwards–less improved and understood, more degraded and bypassed. Foucault's *L'histoire de la folie* (Foucault 1961), translated as *Madness and Civilization* (Foucault 1965), supposed that a relatively common chatter and traffic between "madness" and "reason", occurring chaotically across the landscapes of Medieval Europe, was gradually replaced, under Enlightenment logics of Reason capturing Unreason, by expert discourses of medicine, psychiatry and (later) psychoanalysis which only listened to themselves–to their own self-serious pronouncements–rather than to what the "mad" (now rebranded as the mentally ill, the psychotic, the hysteric, and so on) might *really* be saying about their own lifeworlds. There are multiple complications with the substance of Foucault's mammoth anti-progressivist history (Philo 2013), but it cannot be denied that Foucault's retelling of the famous "reforms" instigated by Pinel in Paris or the Tukes of York has forever shaken up simplistic assumptions about a grand triumph of humanitarianism over oppression, of care over control.

Particularly provocative (for the current volume) is his scathing critique of the experiment with a supposedly benign *moral treatment* furthered by Old William Tuke and his family at the so-called York Retreat, a large country-house set in attractive countryside several miles from the northern English city of York, wherein "moral" versions of architecture (creating a home-like feel) and location (rustic, calming, therapeutic) were deliberately manipulated to ostensibly benevolent ends. For Foucault, however, the result was not care-full liberation but a gigantic "moral" control where "fear [was] addressed to the invalid [the mental 'patient'] directly, not by instruments but in speech, ...

marking out and glorifying a region of simple responsibility where any manifestation of madness will be linked to punishment" (Foucault 1965, 246). More narrowly and indeed geographically, the design was "to constitute for [the patient] a *milieu* where, far from being protected, he [*sic.*] will be kept in perpetual anxiety, ceaselessly threatened by [l]aw and [t]ransgression" (245). The upshot was arguably to stage an abuse even more profound than abandonment in the workhouse cellar, since "the mad" were no longer allowed to be "mad" but had to learn to be sane (which, in Foucault's book, was precisely not the same as being cured). Elsewhere, I have discussed at length the "moral geographies" of the York Retreat and their unparalleled influence in the transformation of the spaces, internal and external, of lunatic asylum provision in nineteenth-century England and Wales (Philo 2004, esp. Chapt. 6), agreeing with Foucault that such geographies have to be interpreted as technologies of (a "soft") social control.

There are many caveats to be introduced–and thunderous disputes to be anatomised between Foucault and his aghast critics of a more progressivist bent (Philo 2004, esp. Chapt. 2)–and Spierenburg's caution that "the reaction against ... optimism [about progress] went too far in the other direction" (Spierenburg 1984, 6) probably should be applied to Foucault's more polemical manoeuvres (including his assault on the Tukes and their Retreat). Even so, post-Foucault the dialectic of care and control becomes an unavoidable feature on the map of social-welfare institutional studies, so that even an ardent anti-Foucauldian such as Roy Porter, in his final book *Madness: A Brief History*, has to engage with Foucault's critical stance in its balance-sheet of modern psychiatry's gains and losses (Porter 2002, esp. 3-7, Chapt. 9). Importantly too, Foucault's own intellectual evolution saw him rework the essentially negative view of control contained in *Madness and Civilization*, arriving at a more sophisticated conceptualisation of power as often operating not repressively but "productively", generatively, making things happen rather than merely stopping them. Such is the lens on power, control and discipline that arises in his text *Discipline and Punish* (Foucault 1977, Philo 2001), ostensibly tracing "the birth of the prison", but actually showing how a new calculus of modern disciplinary power, dependent on multiple spatial tactics ('the art of distributions') for which Jeremy Bentham's *Panopticon* was but one model, became effective in the production of "docile bodies" and disciplined subjects. The Tukes' moral geographies can readily be recast through this lens, as in effect Foucault did himself in his little-known *Psychiatric Power* (lectures 1973-1974; Foucault 2006) when revisiting and amplifying his claims about nineteenth-century asylums (and psychiatry and psychoanalysis) through the optic of *Discipline and Punish* (Philo 2007, 2012, 2013). Seen in this light, care and control really do fuse together–care demands control, control demands care–to the point where it becomes hard to tell where one ends and the other begins; and such a fusion, of course, is what the likes of Pimbo (Unwin) took as entirely "natural", right, beyond question. Such a fusion, as channelled through architectural forms, is of course also the fulcrum of the philosophically-charged conversation between Gunnar Olsson and Martin Gren which commences this volume. To my mind, then, any properly constituted inquiry into "caring architecture" must of necessity also be an inquiry into "controlling architecture", where it becomes a key question as to precisely how the care proceeds through exerting control while the control succeeds through offering care (and how, of course, space is woven throughout this difficult hybrid mixture).

Structure and play, again

> There are ... many dangers in monumentalising spacing, turning it into some kind of solid building and thereby effacing its strange movements, arresting and domesticating them by gathering them together. ... [A]rchitecture is, in the end, a certain effect of the pervasive, ongoing and irresolvable internal conflict that covertly entangles all the lines it appears to so unproblematically draw. Architecture is no more than the strategic effect of the suppression of internal contradiction. It is not simply a mechanism that represses certain things. Rather, it is the very mark of repression. (Wigley 1993, 207-208, 209)

This statement comes from an advanced scoping of the margins between the disciplinary field of architecture and the Derridean critical theory of deconstruction, one where the author, Mark Wigley (1993), an academic architect, investigates the architectural metaphors, allusions and figures present within deconstructive discourse–chiefly Jacques Derrida's own writings–in part as the basis for a deconstruction of deconstruction. In the statement he underlines how architecture, as both idea and practice, often solidifies into a "monument", a "solid building", that cannot but effect a stabilising and homogenising of the ingredients comprising its immediate spaces, ossifying forms rather than releasing "spacings" (as processes of using, feeling and contesting spaces by all manner of agents). As such, architecture effaces movements, domesticates inhabitations and suppresses contradictions, "the very mark of repression", an intriguing claim given remarks above about needing, with Foucault, to think beyond repression when contemplating the play of care and control. Here Wigley ponders how the lines that architects draw on their blueprints almost inevitably slip into clunky realities, the edifices that endure, the underlying will being to drive apart the "stuff" of the world that, in practice and despite the architect, retains its own urges to re-entangle in ways mocking of the controlling orders issued from the drafting table. Put like this, of course, Wigley revisits a fairly familiar terrain of debate for architectural critics of various hues, including architectural geographers (eg. Kraftl 2010, Kraftl and Adey 2008, Jacobs and Merriman 2011), who suppose that the study of architecture should attend less to the *a priori* blueprints (the sharply drawn lines, boundaries and barriers on paper or screen) and more to the lived, multi-sensual experience of people dwelling in the buildings concerned (whose everyday spatial occupations may "crazy up" the lines, nurturing lively spacings rather than acquiescing in dead spaces: see also Yaneva's afterword to this volume). Put like this too, Wigley's thinking dovetails with concerns voiced in the Olsson-Gren conversation, unsurprisingly perhaps given that over the years Olsson has consistently deconstructed the "lines of power" (Olsson 1991) that emanate from the setting of boundaries in thought, word and deed, as well as investigating the complex, power-laden "dialectics of form and process".

Central to the current volume is precisely this tension between architectural forms, with their in-built visions of usage, order, control and maybe programmes of care, and their more ambiguous, changeable and possibly non-compliant inhabitation. In their introduction, Catharina Nord and Ebba Högström describe institutions as "perhaps the most difficult of architectures", where "difficult" clearly means the blocky, hard-edged materiality of institutional spaces, usually shaped by the impulses of coercive power, and they acknowledge the difficulty of stirring an ethics of care–of healing, of kindness–into such inflexible spaces. They draw upon the non-representational sensibilities of contemporary human geography (Anderson and Harrison 2010b) to envisage alternative versions of *architectural geography*, ones resisting the ossification suggested by the Wigley quotation, and, crucially, proposing that successful instances of institution-based care are less likely to arrive from pre-programmed care plans (and care spaces) than from more *ad hoc* "tinkering" in the lived grain of the spaces involved (Mol, Moser, and Pols 2010). Meanwhile, in her own chapter Högström (Chapt. 7) proceeds with a poststructural conception of "spacing", akin to Derrida and refracted through Gilles Deleuze and Felix Guattari, the ambition being to craft "understandings of spaces as 'doings' and 'differentials', as events and spacings." Moreover, she reckons that the SMHC was designed by psychiatrists, in dialogue with architects, who, if not being directly influenced by such conceptually charged ways of thinking space, still possessed an acute sense of wanting to create a series of spatial scenes in the facility which, in their relative *in*determinacy freed from status hierarchies or functional over-specification, could be used multiply, caringly and care-fully, by both staff and patients. Spaces of "non-directed encounter", open-access spaces, variable spatial niches and the like: all of these elements featured in the architectural story of the SMHC, even as they sometimes met with caution and opposition for not being determined or constrained enough.[1]

The two chapters on assisted living for older people work within this tension between architecture as pre-scripted *territory* and architecture as ambiguously, unpredictably lived-in spaces (or spacings). Andersson's chapter (Chapt. 6) identifies "an underlying conflict between how architecture is conceived and perceived, on the one hand, and how it is lived, on the other"; thereby contrasting the "normative usability" expectations of the design process with the messiness of actual "user-environment interaction", here leading to the under-utilisation of common spaces within assisted living complexes and an apparent retreat into privatised existence in individual rooms. Borrowing from Deleuze and Guattari's concept of *stratum*, an *assemblage* stabilised through "an imposed statistical order of connections and successions", Nord (Chapt. 3) talks of "stratum architecture" as architectural forms sedimented across the centuries by repeating essentially the same building designs, illustrated in her chapter by "an unbroken design chain" of caring facilities for the elderly infirm traceable back to fifteenth-century English almshouses. At the heart of such designs is the common space examined by Andersson, one designated for the pursuit of "community and fellowship", reflecting a largely unspoken "care" assumption that elderly infirm residents benefit from engaging in collective being-and-doing with each other. As Nord explains, such an archaic spatial form leads to residents of today's assisted living complexes in Sweden having smaller private rooms than would otherwise be the case, negatively affecting the quality of life for some individuals and couples, and requiring on-the-job tinkering with caring practices in cases where individuals resist being communal or sociable. For Nord, adopting a cautiously optimistic tone, the upshot is "vague caring practices" that "deterritorialise old truths", suggesting possible new caring spaces even within uncaring architectures.

Mention has already been made of Severinsson's chapter (Chapt. 2) and her insistence on the rehabilitative value for troubled teenagers of under-specified, non-directive spaces, in which regard her emphasis on lessening "structure"–on allowing a certain "vagueness" to reign, even in an old rural brick hospital now reused for residential care, as a resource for avoiding stigmatisation or escalation of residents' troubled behaviour–particularly parallels the analysis from Högström. The references to "vagueness" by both Nord and Severinsson are significant, since they tie in with the explicit theorisation of "spatial vagueness" which is the hinge of the chapter by Erling Björgvinsson and Gunnar Sandin (Chapt. 1), rooted in qualitative and ethnomethodological research with patients on a nephrology ward, where the key discovery is that the most appreciated institutional spaces are ones characterised by "vague" or "plastic" specifications of how they might be used and experienced. Standing in near-polar opposition to conventional architectural discourses, where expectations of success lie in precise translations from abstract plan to occupied building, a heretical counter-position emerges which is prepared to countenance under-specification, weak coding and the possibility that things will work out entirely otherwise in how people dwell in–care for and about; tinker with; resist, rework, reuse–the spaces concerned. When Albena Yaneva, in her lovely concluding comments to this volume, suggests that "a caring building is never a stable container", perhaps the implication is that it should *never* be a stable container, but rather always ready-made with possibilities for "many different trials, experiments and adjustments of objects and subjects". At its extreme, this thinking is to contemplate the end of control, the death of the architect and other professional experts, a new anarchistic politics of spacing, and maybe the advent of a genuinely post-institutional age. More modestly, though, it is perhaps to envisage a new play between care and control, where both are complexly distributed rather than centralised in singular institutional authorities, and where control is always care-fully exerted and care leaks beyond complete control. It is to allow play into structure, albeit a play which is deadly serious about ensuring that institutional architectural space for troubled and troublesome humans escapes from the worst excesses of both the institutional and the architectural. Such, arguably, is perhaps the principal clarion-call sounding from this excellent collection of essays.

Notes

[1] I might wish to query certain aspects of this emphasis on 'spatial vagueness' were it to be extrapolated into the claim that *places* do not matter to, say, people with mental health problems. At various moments in my own (co-)writing (eg. Parr 1999, 2006, Philo and Parr 1995, Parr, Philo, and Burns 2003), I stress that feeling 'placed' in the world, 'belonging' somewhere identifiable within clear spatial limits, *can* actually be extremely helpful for people with mental health problems who may often feel dangerously unplaced, dislocated and unbounded. Such a place can even be an old asylum, its buildings and grounds, notwithstanding the entirely appropriate critiques that the anti-psychiatrists and psychiatric survivor movements direct at 'closed spaces' where inmates are deprived of their liberty and often open to sustained abuse. There is a thorny nest of issues here, ones highly relevant to the current volume.

CHAPTER ONE

HOSPITALISATION AND SPATIAL VAGUENESS: PATIENTS' SENSE OF PLASTICITY IN A CARE ENVIRONMENT

ERLING BJÖRGVINSSON AND GUNNAR SANDIN

Hospitalisation and the making of space

In order to acquire a sense of belonging and to resist what in the philosophy of social space has been called *spatial domination* (Lefebvre 1991), i.e. the imposition of foreign ordering principles upon lived space, people tend to develop emancipatory ways of managing their socio-spatial circumstances (Rancière 2005). Such emancipatory spatial production can be described in terms of techniques for appropriating space, but also in terms of the active ability to give and take shape. The latter approach is used in this chapter to reflect on how patients manoeuvre the sense of vagueness in an interior hospital space.

The emancipatory appropriation of space, the desire to make personal aesthetic adjustments and the manoeuvring of one's mobility are all dimensions of making one's daily space more satisfactory or, as it were, are elements of the plasticity of giving and taking form (Malabou 2010). These components of spatial production are defined relationally and cannot be fully provided by programmed or pre-existing architectural functions, such as private room solutions, transit areas, semi-public common spaces in wards and rooms dedicated to the operation of equipment. In architectural definitions of space, and perhaps especially in the precarious and clinical spaces that hospitals provide, a design is often presented and adhered to throughout construction and use, as generalised recurring solutions. These solutions are often intended to be lasting and are achieved at great cost, but despite efforts to provide rooms with clear and explicitly defined functions, spaces within hospitals inevitably also produce a sense of vagueness (Miller 2006), especially from the point of view of patients trying to make these into their own space. The basic hypothesis examined in this chapter is that the appearance of vagueness must inevitably arise, but that there are different types of vagueness. In an investigation into patients' handling of hospital space which this chapter builds upon (Björgvinsson and Sandin 2015), we found that a certain measure of vagueness re-appeared as an issue in the making and changing of possible conditions for movement and socio-spatial self-positioning. In accordance with that and in a reflection on theoretical perspectives on spatial appropriation and subjectivity production, there is a need for vagueness and plasticity as concepts to be further theorised. Moreover, the dual experience of vagueness (to obstruct or to allow action) and the recognition of the reciprocal qualities of plasticity (to give and take shape) need to find ways into a practice- and design-orientated discourse of space, in the present case with specific attention to hospital space.

Vagueness and the plasticity of spatial appropriation

In an environmental study with sociological and psychological implications, Korosec-Serfaty (1973) made an early interpretation and application of Henri Lefebvre's philosophy of everyday spatial production and presented a tangible view on the appropriation of space. In its summarising conciseness, this view could be seen as forecasting later theorisation on how architectural and urban space is accessed, assimilated and protected. In line with Lefebvre, but in a more applied manner, Korosec-Serfaty viewed appropriation not as an act of depriving somebody else of something, but as an act of internalising the spatial circumstances in which one is situated. Following analysis of spontaneous modes of spatial production, such as the appropriative and emancipatory actions taken when someone first moves into a new apartment or adjusts to a renovated public square, Korosec-Serfaty (1973) concluded that such appropriative production of space occurs in acts of making territorial delimitation of a place. These acts include inviting other people to rooms made for living, using forbidden zones, personalisation through the display of objects and partial destruction of material elements. She described several modes of making a place into one's own for a sense of belonging, including overturning or even destroying the existing spatial order. In this regard, Korosec-Serfaty and her contemporary, Erving Goffman, could be said to be forerunners when dealing with the self-regulation of social frameworks tied to situational frames. In this line of thought, Goffman's (1986) basic idea was that members of a particular group or society actively produce frameworks and shared belief systems. Frameworks reflect how people bring into any situation a set of expectations and interpretive schemes guiding how a situation should be interpreted and enacted. Any encounter therefore carries constraints where the participants take on pre-ordained roles, producing what Goffman calls "frame spaces". In a hospital context, it is possible to forecast and recognise roles such as diagnostician, healer, announcer, speaker, questioner and nurse that are allocated to doctors and nurses, whereas roles such as nursed, healed, palliated, listener, overhearer are allocated to patients. Such framework constraints and role structures are to some extent modified in intersubjective and successively emerging framing of more specific activities. At times, Goffman acknowledges, a situation should be understood or defined as unclear, and thus as producing frame ambiguity. On the whole, however, Goffman focuses on how individuals interpret frames and less on how frames are strategically used to produce new signification, anticipatory structures and action, in order to reframe frameworks and frame spaces (Baker 2006). Korosec-Serfaty, on the other hand, focuses precisely on such productive resistance, realised through materially and spatially conditioned activities.

In the precarious, sometimes urgent or even life-or-death situation that may be part of a patient's medical care, but also in the more routine-governed rehabilitating stay in hospital, the normal personal control of space is disturbed. It is replaced by fragmentary attempts by the individual to regain a sense of unscattered self. Such attempts can be described in terms of "plasticity", or the giving and receiving of form, as defined by Catherine Malabou. According to that author, plasticity can be seen as a general force of adaptive formation, general because it applies to formation in several fields: philosophy, neurology, translation, art, writing, etc. (Malabou 2010). Plasticity is a principle of formation resulting in wholeness as well as destruction (Malabou 2012). In a reflection, explicitly on hospitalisation, and more precisely on Merleau-Ponty's (1962) example of how patients may lose a sense of "plasticity" or the capacity to retain wholeness in their hospitalised and thus unfamiliar perception of the world, Malabou (2015, 17) claims that a state of illness tends to create a more scattered state of mind and leaves patients without a grounded sense of self and autonomy. A hospital patient deals with several losses at the same time, for instance being clothed in borrowed, oversized hospital garb forces the patient to deal not only with the disease, but also with an altered identity of "looking like nothing" (Malabou 2012, 71). Losing the sense of being able to achieve and give form in a given situation thus becomes a disturbance in the relationship between a subject and their environment. It is a disturbance that the perceiver (the patient) tries to overcome, seemingly by default. As regards recovery, it is not a far-fetched thought that the environment and its possibility to meet the patient's perceptual needs regarding expectations of what the environment ought to contain in terms of recognisable elements, but also the patient's need to sense that the capacity to perceive is in their own control, is of great importance. In light of this view, architectural and clinical and care thinking could be required to create a hospital space not only through a set of mono-functional demands, but also by imagining the complexity of this reciprocal relationship between environment and patients' need for a "plastic" spatial condition. The necessity of plastic existence suggests that thinking about hospital spaces requires rethinking of the habit of installing specific clinical or aesthetic functions, but it consequently also opens the way for discussion on the necessary presence of a certain type of environmental vagueness. In the study about patients' spatial and aesthetic preferences (Björgvinsson and Sandin 2015), we showed that the issue of spatial vagueness is linked to other issues, such as where the patient must stay, can move, should put their things etc., according to explicit but also sensed or even subjectively fabricated rules of manoeuvring. This is due to impositions caused by the environment. During hospitalisation, the mechanisms of simultaneous reading, forming and destroying the meaning of space become particularly articulated because of the sense of precariousness tied to being ill, being in the custody of unknown caregivers and at the same time living physically on unknown grounds.

From the point of view of logical reasoning, vagueness has traditionally been thought of as a borderline phenomenon that remains resistant to investigation, or representing a case where it is impossible to judge whether certain conditions are included or not in what is investigated (Sorensen 2001). As Sorensen (2012) points out, Charles Peirce, in an entry about "vague" in the 1902 *Dictionary of Philosophy and Psychology*, saw this ambiguous state of matter not as a logical annoyance, but as something that tells us what reality–and talking about reality–is all about (Peirce 1902, 748). Floyd Merrell (1996) reflected on Peirce's distinction between "generality" and "vagueness" as two fundamental elements of the indeterminacy of reality; both imply a necessary incompleteness in how people interpret actual things, but generality, as a concept, fails at "taking in a finite world", whereas vagueness at least "allows for a picking and choosing of possibilities" without presenting a finished whole. Vagueness can be seen as the troubling condition in which people try to bring some kind of order to a given circumstance. Even if vagueness is perhaps most often, particularly in rational situations, seen as a problem where space or information causes inexact use of terms or directives, it can also be seen as the condition where there is enough room for making personal or unplanned manoeuvres. Miller (2006) reflects on the problematic side of vagueness as causing disorientation, but also points, more positively, to the anti-essentialism, heterogeneity and temporality of spatial vagueness. This is in accordance with its conceptualisation in space theory by Massey

(2005) and in the space-orientated philosophy of Deleuze and Guattari (1986), where vagueness is a "generative possibility" to handle with care, rather than a problem to be solved. Vagueness, in this sense, allows for intersubjective negotiation where the subjective standpoints and identities are simultaneously transformed, as negotiation proceeds, in a manner reminiscent of Goffman's re-framing of frameworks (Baker 2006). Between the outer nodes in the logical dichotomy of "clear" and "vague", people create their own semi-ambiguous "modalities" of place (Sandin 2003), in that they sense that for instance they must, may or want to move in specific ways within a place, thus shaping more nuanced place categories.

In the present analysis, we suggest that spatial vagueness and the plasticity of spatial appropriation can productively work together to understand how patients interpret conditions they face and the space of action they identify and perform in acts of obliteration and simultaneous reconfiguration of "their" space.

Studies of vagueness-related issues in hospital space

Within the specific domain of hospital architecture and in studies of what it can offer, the notion of vagueness has been addressed only sparsely and completely without comprehension when it comes to the spectrum of roles it can play. Structured studies conducted within the field of environmental psychology have taken an interest in the particular sense of vagueness that can be part of spatial orientation, mobility and way finding (Ulrich et al. 2004). However, in most of these studies the focus has been on how to eliminate ambiguity, for instance as part of improving understanding of movement (Carpman, Grant, and Simmons 1993), or, quite pragmatically, reducing (the cost of) direction giving by medical staff (Zimring 1990). Some studies have pointed out the role of materiality, for example how being fooled by the physical space can lead to interpretation of it as unsafe, which is then seen as a form, or a stage, of spatial vagueness. For instance, Douglas and Douglas (2004) describe how patients interpreted reflection from shining floors as wet floors, which made them uneasy about leaving their beds to go to the bathroom.

Much of the research on patient perspectives in healthcare environments, especially in the domain of clinical or environmental psychology, is carried out in controlled experimental settings (Douglas and Douglas 2004, Nanda, Eisen, and Baladandayuthapani 2008, Walch et al. 2005, Ulrich 2001, 2006), while ethnographic observation is rarer. Structured or experimental types of observation usually do not allow patient's preferences to appear as: 1) situated in space instead of in relation to controlled image-based presentations; 2) *ad hoc* instead of temporally controlled sequences; 3) categorically undetermined as opposed to theoretically pre-categorised; 4) pointed out, formulated and discussed by the patients themselves. In a study of three patients' experience of spatial production during a limited stay on a nephrology ward (Björgvinsson and Sandin 2015), we asked ourselves how we could refrain from structured categorisation, and as a consequence we designed the interviews and gathering of information in such a way that the plasticity of the experienced space qualities and the preferences stated by the patients could be discussed between us, the patients and the staff on the ward. The study emphasised the creative and emancipatory aspects of spatial production and furthermore, addressed these aspects in a broad view of aesthetics, i.e. without confining them to the experience of experimentally isolated qualities of decoration, artworks or styled interior design.

A research design for investigating spatial preferences

A central component of our qualitative and ethnomethodological method was to gain an understanding of spatial preferences and everyday manoeuvres and methods created by patients when negotiating their spatial order. Our study was based on personal observations by the three patients and photographs they took during their stay on the nephrology ward. This was followed by a shared discussion of the patients' photographs and observations, between patients, staff and us researchers. Certain findings from these conversations were then categorised, presented, and discussed once more in the presence of the patients, ward staff and other physicians of various ranks within the nephrology department at the hospital.

The ward chosen for the study was of a common type in Swedish hospitals (and in large parts of the world where there is sufficient capital to invest in specific architecture for institutional medical care) which means that also the interior design and type of spatial layout, as well as the care of mixed patient groups, were of a form quite common in specialist and general wards. One woman and two men, aged between 45 and 56 years, participated. Through the rich accounts given by these three patients, we could gain insights and successively develop our analytical categories. The patients' observations showed considerable similarities, but also differences, in their experience, allowing us to gain a rich and complex view of their spatial production through only a few accounts. The length of their stay and their state of health (allowing participation), were issues taken into consideration. Patients staying a few weeks were chosen because they had more than fleeting experience of the ward, but also because they had not yet established a relationship to the ward as their "home" or primary place of living.

As an effect of how the patients' spatial preferences were expressed in photos taken, in stories told and in conversations held, it immediately became clear that much attention and energy during hospitalisation is devoted to understanding the vagueness related to mobility and the regulation of one's own spatial situation. In what follows, we provide an account of how this spatial vagueness relates to the plasticity of acts of appropriation.

Modes of coping with spatial vagueness

It is hardly surprising that patients in hospitals invest significantly in constructing private zones and that at times they find it difficult to do so. Even as patients perceive the spatially pre-existing regime/order/ programme expected to govern their stay in hospital, they also find ways of negotiating these norms–and at times they fail to do so. Their spatial experience thus represents a negotiation between normative programmes and their own personal needs and desires. Below we describe the four categories that emerged as a result of our investigation, which can be summed up as room-making, medial expansion, intrusions by others and familiarity.

Private and semi-private room making

One category of spatial production that emerged from our study involved different modes of private and semi-private room making. It is well known that most patients wish to have a private room and that they dislike being frequently moved around in the hospital (Ulrich et al. 2004). Despite recent ambitions to realise those wishes architectonically, many patients still share rooms, which at times forces them to seek or create private partitions of space elsewhere within the facilities for the sake of being alone, or for social gathering on their terms. This spontaneous production of temporary private (and social) space within the shared environment emerges mainly due to lack of privacy and confidentiality in the existing rooms (Barlas et al. 2001). A less acknowledged type of space making occurs when patients wish to create their own rooms within other shared spaces on the ward, such as in the lunchroom, kitchenette, coffee room and lounge.

The atmosphere of shared patient rooms is easily disturbed and attempts to arrange social activities, such as visits from relatives or friends, may therefore be regarded as most conveniently conducted elsewhere. At the same time, patients report how difficult it can be to be forced to scout for shared rooms that can be temporarily turned into a more private setting hosting family and patient together, precisely because of the official status of such rooms as shareable. Making an officially shared space into a temporary private space is thus subsumed under the main programming and such spontaneous production of space thus risks being experienced as a trespass or even a shameful breach of etiquette and the normative behaviour of such spaces. Furthermore, it may be perceived as possible to achieve only through the necessary act of breaking an institutional rule, which would further increase the laborious aspect of this particular type of private place making.

The kitchenette on the ward in our study was programmed as a shared space. Thus, as one patient in the study explained, he did not realise initially that he could create a minor space of his own within it. However, when he was granted his own partition for storing private medicine and food within the shared spatial order and could use it for his own needs, the space became more positively described by the patient, who expressed this as an increase in autonomy on the ward, leading to a sense of well-being. The patient noted that this kind of spatial production was a privilege rather than a spatial arrangement or activity that he had a normal right to or could expect to be provided by the hospital.

Spatial expansion and sheltering through mediation

Rooms that do not have the stated function of retreat can nonetheless be seen as temporarily providing escape and helping patients to forget their hospitalisation. One such example reported in our study was the shower room, which could be populated with personal things (toiletries) and thus gave a temporary appearance of being private space (Fig. 1.1). While this production of an "oasis" was hampered by the presence of other patients' possessions and use of the shower room by staff for temporary storage, with objects that had to be cleared away before the temporary private sense of place could be created, it was perceived as a space for escape and retreat. Over an extended period, this space was shared by providing room for several needs, thus also signalling to others a needed type of functional vagueness.

Two of the patients used media to give their shared rooms a private character and a possibility to shut out their immediate surroundings while connecting to their social worlds outside the hospital. Media devices (tablets and the like) thus had the function of altering the spatial scope and order. In this regard, various media provided considerable plasticity that simultaneously formed and destroyed prevailing spatial orders. Headphones in particular signalled that a patient did not want to be disturbed, thus creating a transparent private chamber, a reclusive bubble. Photographs from the patient's home expanded the meaning of the room by connecting to familiar remote spaces, thus stimulating the sense of social relations. In this way media, whether analogue and passive and thus working by way of association, or networked and literally plugged into the networks of the life outside, had the function of de-hospitalising and normalising patients' stay.

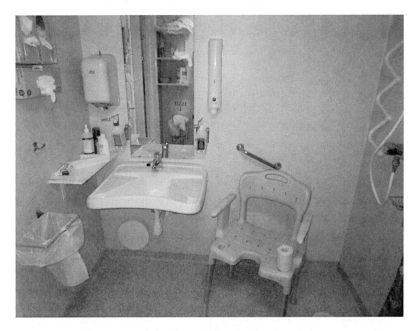

Fig. 1.1. A patient reported that he could make the shared shower room into a temporary private and personal space for retreat, even if the production of such a space was made more difficult by the presence of other patients' toiletries. Photo copyright: Erling Björgvinsson and Gunnar Sandin. Photographed by contracted anonymous patient.

The patients experienced considerable differences between being visited and visiting. Leaving the ward–going to the main hall and especially to the kiosk in the foyer at the main entrance–was experienced as awkward, even shameful. Spaces readily open and accessible to the general public were perceived as first and foremost belonging to the public and only secondarily as belonging to the patients. The ward, and in particular the patients' bedrooms, were considered more suitable to host the appearance and role of being a patient. Hence, patients found it considerably more acceptable if they would have local access to "external" services and activities, such as having a kiosk wagon come to the ward, rather than having to leave the ward. Such close but still "external" services would become part of the territory where the patients had more control of their daily affairs.

Professional intrusions related to number of patients

Various forms of meeting places were considered positive by the patients in our study, including rooms for interactions: patient-patient, patient-nurse, patient-nursing aide or patient-doctor. Sharing experiences with others was considered positive, including any possibility for staff to have time and space to support the exchange of a few words on a personal or a more common level. Even sample taking, which is seldom considered enjoyable or as something to look forward to, was in one case considered a positive break from unexciting days and hours. However, in line with earlier studies on involuntary intrusion (Barlas et al. 2001), the presence of staff and attention from the staff were not always considered positive in our study, as the patients reported how the medical and care staff intruded into their lives. One patient stated while he had the right not to be entangled with the staff's workload or the state of other patients, he was involuntarily forced to be involved, given that the alarm system pierces (the soundscape of) the whole ward. The abrupt change in auditory conditions created by alarms caused the patient to guess the level of work facing the staff or the state of health of the patient causing the alarm.

Several statements showed, as found in other investigations (Ulrich et al. 2004), that shared bedrooms are problematic in ways that not only concern direct patient-patient relations. For example, it was stated by the interviewees that traffic and presence of staff and visitors made them feel as though their bed was in a corridor. In other words, the corridor function (of facilitating transport rather than direct attention towards patients) extended into the patients' room. This in turn had the effect that some patients were unwillingly involved in the treatment of other patients. In some extended periods, such involvement can become explicit, for example, when confused dementia patients cannot tell the difference between staff and patients. However, the shared room concept does not always have to be replaced by a single-room concept, a solution often favoured today in research and in the practice of the hospital design that can afford it. One of the patients in our study suggested for instance that spatial separation within the shared room domain between dementia patients and other patients would significantly increase the sense of privacy. Another patient suggested a simple logistical move: that the patient needing the most care should simply be placed closest to the door, which would give the other patients an increased sense of having a space of their own. One alternative to the preferred single-bedroom solution might thus be to have flexible room logistics, for instance, if possible, by allowing one bed to remain empty as long as possible in rooms with several beds. Another alternative could be to make unwanted over-hearing more difficult with sound-absorbing curtains. Such solutions, forwarded as ideas by the patients in our study, would increase the sense of plasticity in the spatial environment.

Aesthetic effects: decoration, homeliness and unfamiliarity

Certain elements of space are often denoted as specifically aesthetic. These include lighting, window views, colouring and art, which have received considerable attention within evidence-based studies of patients' perspectives on hospital architecture (Ulrich 2006). In our study, these elements received only limited attention from the patients, even though the questionnaire asked what the patients "like" and "prefer". As some of the patients' comments showed, aesthetic decoration was to some degree connected to the notion of the home and homeliness. Furthermore, certain colours, greenery and sounds of nature were described as associated with pleasure, cosiness or homeliness. However, it was not explicitly stated that they had a calming effect (Fig. 1.2), even if the attribute "cosy" could be understood as closely associated with calm and relaxed atmospheres. Nevertheless, it was explicitly expressed by all participants in the study that the hospital should not aim for a homely feeling. The patients were quite clear about not wanting the hospital to become a second home. Too much homeliness, they explained, would increase their sense of not being able to build their own spatial order–their own home place aesthetics–and this could lead to an oppressive sense of entrapment and prolonged stay, instead of a healing hospitalisation.

A traditional view regarding personal appropriation of space is that the home, as an ideal space, satisfies people's sense of corporeal belonging, as well as their "aesthetic-political aspiration" (Tuan 1991, 102). On the other hand, a home can also be oppressive, as Cresswell (2004) notes in reference to Rose (1993), and Martin and Mohanty (1986). Conversely, a non-home like a highway café or a workplace can for some people contain as much placeness and homeliness as a traditional home or home-like architecture (Sandin 2003). Regardless of the kind of actual place that allows a relaxed or "home-like" relationship, the sense of plasticity tied to a relaxed perceptual ability appeared in our study not only to act as factual spatial appropriation, but was also linked to the patients' sense of having perceptual control due to the familiarity of decorative qualities. Creswell points out that homelessness is not simply a being without a home, but can be a "disconnection from a particular form of place" or an existential "displacement" that "is perhaps even more fundamental than being without shelter" (Cresswell 2004, 111, 115). Malabou (2015) also points out how patients, although physically sheltered in a hospital, may feel existentially scattered, lacking autonomy and a sense of wholeness.

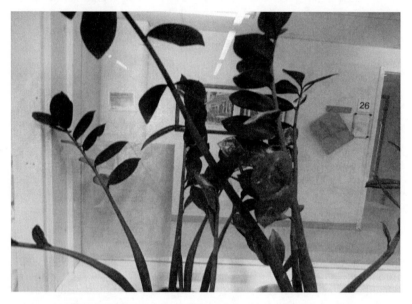

Fig. 1.2. Plants, colours and artworks are appreciated as reducing the sterile aspects of the hospital environment, but they are only of marginal interest. The presence of such elements, according to the patients, should preferably be kept at a modest level in order not to produce too homely a feeling. Photo copyright: Erling Björgvinsson and Gunnar Sandin. Photographed by contracted anonymous patient.

In our study, the patients experienced unfamiliarity when there was a gap between the socio-spatial arrangement and their comprehension of it. The difficulty of deciphering or reading an unknown, but much specified, socio-spatial order may create feelings of unease and unnecessary projections/fantasies. For instance, the medical equipment hanging on walls or standing in the patient rooms or in corridors can appear frightening if the patient does not know what it is for. Imbuing things with meaning, in this fuzzy medical environment full of equipment and activities, seems to be a central human impulse, as the absence of meaning can be more uncomfortable than a "wrong" reading. Reading some sort of intentionality and socially constructed framework into spaces, things and activities is simply difficult to refrain from, as emphasised by Goffman (1986).

The perceived health status of other patients in the ward may also trigger uncertainty in a patient's spatial experience. For example, it can be disturbing to have a coughing and hawking patient close by and sharing a space with such a patient can be perceived to be medically unsound and very frightening by a patient susceptible to infection. This can lead to an ambiguous reading of the socio-spatial situation as a whole, making the occurrences on the ward more frightening than they actually are.

Spatial "misreading" of an actual condition is thus clearly not limited to material environmental issues such as the lack of daylight for orientation, the colouring of floors for way-finding or blank surfaces, but also includes (fear of) socio-material configurations related to medical treatment and care.

Having recognised the necessity and complexity of at least certain home-like and recognisable qualities in hospital environments, it is also important to note that aesthetic qualities, to use that term in its broadest sense, cannot be delimited to recognition, just as they cannot be reduced to decoration but must also include transgressive elements (Sandin 2015). The extent to which aesthetic effects have a remedying role to play in hospital space thus remains a disputed issue (Sandin and Ståhl 2011).

Concluding thoughts

Spatial vagueness in an emancipatory orientated place discourse has been ascribed positive and productive values (Lefebvre 1991, Korosec-Serfaty 1973, Malabou 2010, 2012, 2015, Massey 2005, Deleuze and Guattari 1986), while in a more rationalistic hospital architecture research perspective it has been related to disorientation and considered a negative attribute (Ulrich et al. 2004). Thus, the modalities of vagueness are considerable. The plasticity of the state of hospitalisation, i.e. the ability to give as well as receive an unprogrammed change of conditions, was seen to be of great importance in our study. In relation to the scattering effect, but also the useful indeterminacy, of vagueness, it is clear that the way in which space is produced and the partial or whole "solutions" that appear as responding to patients' spatial needs are issues that need to be addressed more actively, in a way where the subject is not reduced to a mere recipient.

Vagueness appears to be an attribute tied to matter and to social bonds, an attribute of a negative and positive kind. Importantly, however, vagueness as a state is always spatially present and experienced differently, depending for instance on the acquaintance with the immediate environment. On the one hand, it can be seen as generating unease when the relationship is unclear, in the

present case between the insufficient physical architectural arrangements and
the patient, between the unknown equipment and the patient, or between the
patient and other patients or members of staff. A patient, especially a newcomer
to a ward, has not learned through practice what these relationships mean, and
a certain amount of vagueness is consequently produced. However, a certain
amount of vagueness is also needed to gain an understanding of what unknown
things, proximities and conditions mean to the patient, and such understanding
cannot be remedied through inscribing into objects, proximity and conditions a
designed message as in functionalist semiotic attempts. Rather, their meaning
arises relationally on the ward, as a multifaceted communication between daily
practice and the handled situation in a complex act of spatial plasticity. A
disturbing type of vagueness appeared in this study, for instance precisely
because a patient had not been sufficiently introduced, or cultured, into these
relations. A too object-centred view on communication, believing that a precise
(socio-material) language conveys the message, does not acknowledge how
meaning is relationally constructed. A welcoming act can to some extent be
eased, but not sufficiently fulfilled, by for instance avoiding unnecessary
exposure to elements that might provoke frightening associations or uncertainty.
A more profound and at the same time more flexible support to acclimatisation
into the environment and its practice happens through interactions with the staff
and other patients and by being allowed to alter the spatial situation.

Apart from various types of frightening vagueness, expressed as gaps in the
interpretation of space and communicational shortcomings, vagueness is also
sensed by patients as necessary, such as when their urge to produce niches of
their own appears as a kind of spatial "medium" for the possibility of re-
creational plasticity to appear. The social reframing of some of the semi-public
areas–the lounge, the patient kitchenette and the coffee room–into temporary
private zones becomes partly possible since these zones are read as actually
having a semi-vague programming, allowing the patients to appropriate them
for personal needs.

However, the possibility to reshape shared spaces like the lounge or the
coffee room into semi-private spaces can at any time be disturbed or dissolved,
which shows that the plasticity of these semi-public spaces works both ways.
As easily as semi-private spaces can be produced, they can be quickly
destroyed. The scouting for semi-private rooms may come about because the
patient rooms are negatively vague, paradoxically sensed as not distinct,
because they are difficult to format on one's own terms, while the formatting
plasticity given by static positions, strange objects and definite interior framing
can be more extensive. The kitchenette's vagueness, for example, if considered
in relation to who can use all its niches, allows for a reshaping that may hold
over an extended period of time, as it is not under constant danger of being

dissolved. The shared shower room, likewise, despite the presence of other patients' possessions, allows for a more profound sense of reshaping than is possible in the kitchenette, since the patient can shut out certain disorder and create the illusion, although only temporary, of having their own private room. In this way, the term vagueness productively points at how meaning making is relationally produced and negotiated. Vagueness here reflects Merrell's (1996, 38) "picking and choosing", and Miller's (2006) anti-essentiality, as more open and creative ways of dealing with space than just aligning with its generalised qualities, even when these qualities–appearing in hospitals for instance as specific functions attributed to single rooms, private bathrooms, window views, good art, etc.–are conceived in the best of design intentions.

We have discussed the fact that patients are actively engaged in producing spatial orders and experiences and that a certain measure of spatial vagueness is needed for this. The fact that patients are more concerned with constructing privacy, sociability, mobility and spatial readability than with decorative dimensions of the hospital environment, is an argument for a more profound appreciation of the plastic possibilities of spatial formation. Acknowledging the importance of plastic aspects of spatial production implies more moderate programming of the physical environment and recognising rather than rejecting patients' need to renegotiate frameworks.

In a theoretical account, we raised the value of pairing vagueness and plasticity. The notion of vagueness helped us identify indeterminate and ambiguous existential conditions tied to the materially and socially constructed space, as identified by the patients in our study. Plasticity and appropriation, on the other hand, were useful concepts for analysing how the patients productively dealt with vagueness through various forms of obliteration and reconfiguring of existing spatial formations. Plasticity, more than appropriation, was seen as the reconfiguring of space in acts of mutual making and unmaking of the circumstances at hand.

In addition to the phenomenological view on perception, where a passive singular subject-patient (Merleau-Ponty 1962) is seen as coping with illness, we acknowledged a subject-patient in line with Malabou (2015, 2012), where the formation of space is actively given and taken. In acknowledgment of the patient's interaction with the hospital environment, its physical objects and the actions of patients and staff, findings expressed by patients themselves revealed that plasticity is a feature of the living formation of meaning, and vagueness is part of the activated dealing with environmental elements. In line with this, we argue for a need to pay attention to the active and disruptive subject, rather than to the passive perceiver/conceiver, in spatial thinking and in the design of space, not least hospital space.

CHAPTER TWO

THE ART STUDIO:
BOTH A STABILISER AND A MOBILISER
IN TRANSLATIONS OF RESIDENTIAL CARE
HOMES FOR TROUBLED TEENAGERS

SUSANNE SEVERINSSON

Residential care homes for troubled teenagers

Residential care homes for troubled teenagers are sometimes described as places for young people acting "mad, bad and sad" (Wright 2009, 288), where the societal task is to put them "back on the right track". In answer to my question of why someone is placed in a residential care home, 14-year-old Jimmy provided an alternative description: "It is because we have not managed in school and we have done a lot of things. Being violent or assaulting people". Causes for a stay can also be described more vaguely, as in 14-year-old Emma's account: "I do not know what I am supposed to get treatment for here. I have seen a psychologist in town two times but he does not work here". In some cases, teenagers living in these care homes may have been victims of child abuse or the children of drug abusers; in other cases, individuals may be described as criminals or offenders; and sometimes both situations apply. Neuropsychiatric diagnoses such as *attention deficit hyperactivity disorder (ADHD)* and *Asperger's* are common and all the resident teenagers have in one way or another been identified as having *social, emotional and behavioural difficulties (SEBD)*. To a certain extent these are teenagers who have not been able to manage their lives and who have been failed by the (lack of) support from the grownups around them.

There are many possible reasons for placement in a residential care home. Regardless of past history, however, it is the individual teenager who has been removed from his or her parents in order to be "transformed" in a new environment. In the residential care home, the teenagers meet staff (humans) and interact with materiality (non-humans), resulting in opportunities for them to accommodate to societal norms. However, these interactions also give the teenagers opportunities to generate resistance against changing their behaviour. This chapter presents a non-representational analysis of interactions around the art room in a residential care home, using *Actor-Network Theory (ANT)* (Callon 1986) and *diffractive reading* (Barad 2007). The chapter examines the fluctuating and stabilising aspects of room and materiality in relation to the "mangle" concept; that is, the dialectic of accommodation and resistance proposed by Pickering (1993). The empirical example, used for illustration, is taken from a study in a residential care home for troubled teenagers–a suitable place for studies of how a network can (try to) transform human agency.

Interventions in residential care homes for troubled teenagers are often described as being conducted within the framework of education and social services, and being situated at an intersection of care, treatment and teaching (Landrum, Tankersley, and Kauffman 2003). The residential care homes combine pedagogic and therapeutic methods in a therapeutic milieu (Willmann 2007); however, the teenagers do not always agree with the methods, adding to an already problematic situation. To be changed or to change oneself is not a simple process. Resident teenagers are not always prepared to accept demands to "behave", perhaps because they believe that other people, such as parents or previous teachers, are responsible for their situation.

Although these teenagers sometimes see no point in adapting to societal norms, at other times they are given new hope and help for their future lives (Severinsson 2010). To tackle resistance on the part of the teenagers, the staff tries to build trust and relationships. In addition, the care home is often framed in a homelike style, in order to facilitate this process and communicate institutional good will. Coercion and compulsion are also constantly apparent and a discourse[1] of discipline is underlined and materialised in the form of locked corridors and simultaneous surveillance. Discourses of medicine and education are also materialised in the architecture, furniture and materials, as well as being mixed with each other in discursive practices (Foucault 1977) in a blurred and sometimes confusing manner (Severinsson, Nord, and Reimers 2015, Severinsson and Nord 2015)

Ambiguous spaces and fluctuating aspects of materiality

Many aspects of care for troubled teenagers are muddled and ambiguous, including how the teenagers are described and how their care spaces are designed. The teenagers are in conflict with themselves, their parents, their schools and the law, and have been transferred to a new place in order to change. On entering this ethnographic field, I sought to identify the kinds of (new) places created to handle undesirable behaviour. I discovered that many different arrangements prevail in this field (Severinsson, Nord, and Reimers 2015). First, the residential care homes established to care for troubled teenagers often reuse (old) places and/or architecture. For example, the buildings used are frequently located out in the countryside and were originally built for some other purpose. In my study, I encountered the reuse of such disparate places as an asylum, a home for people with intellectual disabilities, a sanatorium, a farm and a preschool. Apparently, any large empty building will do as a residential care home; there appears to be no awareness of the importance of architecture in these selections, even though architecture plays an active part in all educational settings (Fenwick and Landri 2012).

Architecture is also important in the everyday residential care of fostered teenagers in need of special education and social, psychological and pedagogic inputs (Severinsson, Nord, and Reimers 2015). The existing architecture of the buildings being reused as residential homes sometimes confuses matters; for example, one of the buildings that used to be a farm still feels like one, even though farming as an activity has long since ended. In other cases, great brick buildings such as former hospitals have a very strong agency when reused as homes, through their faceted institutional character. Wide halls, stairs and corridors play a powerful role even if the care home staff try to transform the environment into an "ordinary home" with bright colours, patterned curtains, potted plants, homelike furniture and other artefacts. The state-provided income for troubled teens makes the use of such buildings possible. However, it can be difficult to see what the residential home is intended to be (and what the staff is trying to transform the setting into) when the previous role of the architecture is still so active. Even for someone like myself, with a background as a social worker, it can be difficult to see at a first glance whether a facility is more of a school, a convalescent home or a family home. Some of these settings reflect what Philo and Pickstone (2009, 653) call an "unpromising configuration"–an institutional setting located in a remote rural area, where unhindered experimentation is possible, leading to the development of situated knowledge that conflicts with mainstream thinking. This institutional ambiguity can create a model that defines the teenager in more than one way.

The ambiguity is reflected by the fragments of and muddled variations on knowledge that are used by the staff. The staff's knowledge is recognisable as originally coming from child experts outside the facility; it includes psychological theories such as behaviourism and psychoanalytical theories, but mixes them and uses them side by side with cognitive and pedagogical theories. Ambiguity and a mixed message are also present in the different types of staff members. For example, in the case of *Sandbacken*, a residential home located in a former hospital, there are few qualified teachers. Most of the staff members are undergraduate care assistants, with a few trained social workers and counsellors. A psychologist occasionally visits to guide the other staff members. And of course, the teenagers themselves, both girls and boys, are part of the situation–all designated with various shortcomings and SEBD, yet distinct individuals. My experience with residential care homes indicates that rooms in the homes are used for different purposes at different times; and that flexibility and negotiations regarding what to do and why are in constant interplay (Severinsson, Nord, and Reimers 2015, Severinsson and Nord 2015).

Sandbacken

The empirical material in this study comes from an ethnographic study of a residential care home, Sandbacken, which lasted for 6 months and was documented through field notes and interviews. Sandbacken is a large, three-storey, 19th-century institutional brick building located in the countryside, which was originally built as a hospital. At the time of my study, the residential care home housed a specialised facility for 20 male and female teenagers, whose parents and schools were unable to handle them. The teenagers ranged from 12 to 16 years of age and had a broad spectrum of social and pedagogical problems. In two Swedish research projects, I have studied where and how care and education are produced in different places, and in what kind of setting troubled teenagers are placed. However, solutions similar to Sandbacken can be found in many countries (Berridge et al. 2008, Landrum, Tankersley, and Kauffman 2003, Willmann 2007).

In the mornings, the teenagers at Sandbacken spent time in a room where they followed activities like those in a school classroom, such as filling in missing words on a worksheet or reading an English text. However, the room itself was not furnished like an ordinary classroom: it had only a few tables, and included a sofa that made the room look rather like a day-room in a hospital–for example, like a room in a psychiatric day-care facility. The high ceiling reinforced this impression. The dining hall at Sandbacken looked like a hotel dining room, with a large table on which a buffet of different dishes was served, while meals were enjoyed at small tables with attractive tablecloths. However, just outside the dining hall a huge staircase provided access to the upper floors, where many doors were locked and infrequently used. This mixed environment created an ambiguous impression and produced faceted perspectives from which to understand the situation. The remote location of Sandbacken, and the fact that it is a privately owned small company with short decision paths, created space for the management and staff to experiment and examine different methods and activities. Thus, residential care for troubled teenagers can be described as a kind of "paradoxical space" (Rose 1993, Spandler 2009, 677) that is, a potentially creative space for alternative practices.

A mangle of resistance and accommodation?

Everyday institutional life in a residential home, with its double societal mission of providing care while also disciplining the troubled teenager, is complex. The configurations of care change quickly, such as in how processes of accommodation and resistance come into play in daily life. This interplay relates to "the dialectic of resistance and accommodation" and the "mangle" concept proposed by Pickering (1993). Pickering suggests that the mangle concept is useful for the production of new scientific knowledge; however, this concept can be used as both a figuration and an analytical tool, as proposed by Jackson (2013).

> Resistance (and accommodation) is at the heart of the struggle between the human and material realms in which each is interactively restructured with respect to the other–in which material agency, scientific knowledge, and human agency and its social contours are all reconfigured at once (Pickering 1993, 585).

Pickering claims that it is difficult to know what is going to happen beforehand in a network; a suggestion that certainly fits the description of a residential care home for troubled teenagers. He and other Actor-Network Theory (ANT) scholars assert that human goals and intentions are constantly transformed, and argue for a decentralised human subject and a decentralised agency (Murdoch 1998, Law 1999, Latour 1984). Jackson (2013, 742) writes that using the mangle concept as an analytical tool makes it possible to depart from a search for the "essential, stable human (and knowledge and experience) of the centre of the inquiry" and embrace the intertwined relations between human and non-human actors. Post-humanistic theories contend that neither human nor non-human actors possess intentionality; rather, intentionality is produced and changed in the interplay between human and non-human agencies (Latour 2005).

Smyth, McInerney, and Fish (2013) argue that it is crucial to consider the socio-material dimension and the affective (relational) aspects of the places to which disadvantaged young people are sent and to focus less on a prescribed curriculum. Studies on the education of troubled teenagers could gain significantly from analyses based on a post-structural perspective, particularly when examining educational disengagement and its complexity (Fenwick and Landri 2012). I started to use ANT as an analytical tool because this theory considers human and non-human actors to be symmetrical. For example, architecture and materials can be given equal consideration in an ANT analysis, and both can be treated as important actors in the network. In ANT, interactions within networks are encompassed by the concept of *translation*. Here, a translation is a process that defines how the interactional situation can be understood, and how appropriate roles and ways to act emerge (Callon 1986). I apply the translation approach in the present analysis in order to study the processes in play at Sandbacken. In such a context, definitions, roles and agency can shift very quickly, especially if actors do not agree on a particular definition of a situation or, in the language of ANT, if the translations are fluctuating and mobile. An ANT analysis allows the simultaneous consideration of a number of actors–in this case, including teenagers, professionals, materials and different environments–and makes it possible to analyse situations from multiple angles at the same time. The analytical focus of the translation approach enables examinations of how the network produces different knowledge and subjectivities. Thus, ANT can be used for the double articulation of a materiality both stabilising a network while simultaneously partaking in mobility and flow.

The network of an art studio is analysed here in terms of translations of humans and materialities. The aim is to investigate how the knowledge and subjectivities fluctuate in different translations of materiality and human actors. A translation can be analysed through the four characteristics described by Callon (1986, 201-208): problematisation, interessement, enrolment and mobilisation. When human and non-human actors in the network come together, one or more *problematisations* come into play; these can be described as the finding out or identification of what is happening. The problems are then formulated and reformulated by negotiations of the *interessements*–that is, the aspects of why a problem is happening and/or what is involved–in order to attach the actors more closely to the network and counteract any resistance to emergent network assignments. The next characteristic, *enrolment*, refers to the ways in which actors invite others or present themselves. The actors are enrolled by each other according to the interessement, and the enrolment designates, to a certain extent, how the actors are perceived. Finally, the characteristic of *mobilisation* refers to what is to be done, and means that actions are taken within a translation. The process that has just been described is not a linear enactment; rather, it lurches and shifts back and forth between the different stages in the translation process.

In translations, designations are not seen as descriptive; instead, they are performative and produce different knowledge and possible subjectivities as well as limiting how the actors are perceived (Youdell 2006, 2011). As Philo and Pickstone (2009) point out, some geographies are so complex and varied that even the use of numerous conceptual and methodological tools is insufficient to explore their complexity, because these tools only take in human aspects and do not value fluctuating relational aspects. The question is: what happens inside this ambiguous space, and how can sense be made of something that seems so fluctuating and faceted? The analysis here illustrates the fluctuating and stabilising aspects of the art studio network as well as how accommodation and resistance (the mangle) come into play. But are the characteristics of Callon enough to understand everything that is going on? In the analysis, I discovered that the spatial and discursive ambiguity existing both inside and outside the art studio played an important role in the network dynamics and involved other human actors and materiality, whether present or not. Because of this openness and vagueness regarding "what", "where" and "why", several possible translations came into play at the same time. The complexity of the situation also attached an important role to the analysis used, as this influences what is possible to "discover". Barad (2007) discusses the impact of the researcher's methods, which define and limit what can be explored. To capture the complexity of the network under study, I used Barad's diffractive methodology in combination with the concept of translation (Callon 1986).

Diffractive reading provided a way to examine several possible understandings of what was happening simultaneously in the art studio, in different layers. I used diffractive reading while analysing the example several times: shifting between different discursive lenses as all of Callon's translation stages shifted as well. The discursive lenses captured the Sandbacken network of pedagogical and methodological approaches in its totality–a network in which different discursive perspectives came into use in everyday life (Severinsson, Nord, and Reimers 2015). Through the use of different discursive lenses, diffractive reading made it possible to display different translations that were being performed simultaneously. The empirical example was read through five different discursive lenses, prompting repeated iterations of my analysis in order to better capture the simultaneity of the different translations instead of having to choose one. Together, the actors involved contribute to the art studio network's creation of a range of alternative translations, each producing a certain agency of what is possible to know and become.

Translations of the art studio network

The setup of the art studio at Sandbacken and its surrounding ambiguous environment–of very wide staircases, high ceilings, stone and brick walls, potted plants, colourful curtains, comfortable sofas and staff called "teachers" yet without a school–give disparate clues as to the purpose of and intentions for the studio. It is a small room in a big building and gives an equivocal impression, which is reinforced by the architecture reflecting Sandbacken's original purpose as a hospital.

An art studio configuration can be found in many places, including mainstream schools, where it can be a classroom for art lessons; hospitals, where it may be designed for recreation or psychiatric art therapy; kindergartens; or private homes, where it is used for professional artwork or simply art play. Upitis (2004) argues that art can engage the whole individual, including the intellect, emotions and physical body. She also problematises the possibility of perceiving art as a holistic activity, such as in schools where the (school) architecture may conflict with the pedagogic goals; for example, in schools that are expected to create responsible democratic citizens in a paradoxically enclosed school environment with high fences and locked doors (Upitis 2004, 21).

In Sandbacken, the pedagogic goals are similarly unclear. The residential care home has the societal task of handling teenagers' undesirable behaviour and of keeping them contained in the home for treatment purposes; however, the objectives of the care and schooling are more nebulous (Severinsson 2015). It was difficult to determine the purpose of the art studio in this study, due to the ambiguous and complex discursive and spatial framing that allowed the studio to be translated in various ways.

The art studio at Sandbacken is a very small space (15 m^2) fitted with wall shelves filled with clay figures, paints, brushes and crayons (Fig. 2.1). Several spatial conditions cause it to be an open and flexible contributor to network processes. The fact that the room is not as large as a normal school classroom is an ambiguous clue to the purpose of its activities. The studio has two windows, but the light is not as good as in a "real" art studio. There is a table in the middle with four chairs around it, and water is available from a tap at a sink. The walls display pictures and paintings produced by the teenagers, although many of these are pre-printed images that have simply been coloured in.

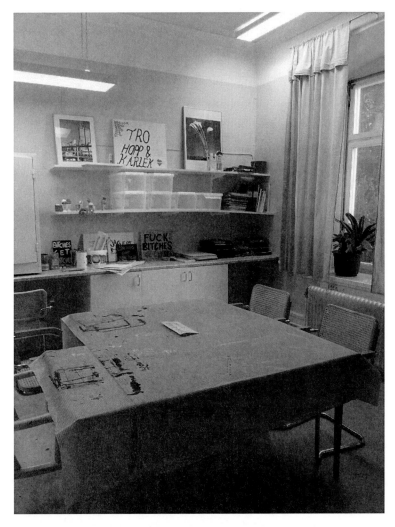

Fig. 2.1. The art studio. Photograph by Susanne Severinsson

It is also ambiguous that the room is used in the mornings, during "school time", but is not housed in a school building and does not accommodate a class. Instead, the teenagers are invited one by one or in pairs to accompany one staff member to the studio. This invitational procedure indicates that the art studio may be considered as a refuge or an oasis of voluntarism in the midst of a residential care home in which teenagers are primarily in an enforced stay. Furthermore, the staff are *not* qualified teachers, psychotherapists or counsellors, but simply have vocational school training as care assistants. My impression was that the teenagers generally did not think of or were not aware of the staff's skills or education. The staff tries to fulfil all the roles of teaching, psychotherapy and counselling, so there is little indication of the specific purpose of their presence in the art studio. The studio is used for different immanent purposes, and sometimes the teenagers and staff have different purposes within it, or no obvious purpose at all (Severinsson, Nord, and Reimers 2015). Every now and then the staff members act as guards, thus appearing in a disciplinary subjectivity.

The human and material actors in the art studio network are products of each other, and different kinds of knowledge and subjectivities emerge in several trajectories of change in which the network interactions are translated differently. This is described by Pickering as the conceptualisation of "temporally emergent phenomena" (Pickering 1993, 561). The analysis below reveals different translations of the same interaction by reading the example through different discursive lenses. As suggested by the mangle concept (Pickering 1993) this variety of translations indicates that the teenagers have the possibility of shifting between translations, rather than making open displays of resistance or accommodating institutional demands.

A teenage girl (15 years old) sits in the art studio with a care assistant and myself (the researcher). When the assistant asks her what she wants to do, she opts to draw. They discuss different types of drawing and painting materials, and the girl chooses crayons. She starts using a black crayon to colour a pre-printed heart image on a sheet. She sighs and then suddenly rips the sheet, crumples it and throws it towards the wastepaper basket. She misses. She now leans back in the chair and looks with blank eyes at the floor in front of her. Nodding at the basket, the care assistant asks: "Is this how you feel?"

The translations of this interaction between a member of staff and a teenage resident shift back and forth in relation to the same materiality; the crayons and paper. An analysis through different discursive lenses reveals (at least) five different translations: (1) an art lesson that changes back and forth into (2) an investigation of the psychosocial situation, (3) psychotherapy, (4) amusement or (5) imprisonment. Each translation enrols the materiality in different ways and designates the staff member and teenager different subjectivities and agencies. Finally, each translation also produces a certain knowledge and mobilises the actors for another translation.

Art lesson

The art lesson occurs when the network is viewed through a pedagogic lens and interpreted as a learning situation. If the network translates the relations as "school", it suggests a lesson in how to draw. The staff member and teenager discuss different types of drawing and painting materials, and the girl chooses crayons. The problematisation in this translation involves the pupil's ignorance (in drawing) and her need to be educated; and the school lesson is the solution. Here, the materials emerge as tools for drawing and learning. The offered subjectivities in this translation are read through the pedagogic lens and the human actors are enrolled as teacher and pupil, even though the pupil is unwilling in this example.

However, when I interviewed the teenagers at Sandbacken, they often chose to apply the pedagogic lens, preferring to see their everyday life as school time because this offered them the possibility of acting as normal teenagers and going to "school" (Severinsson, Nord, and Reimers 2015). Conceptualising this interaction as an art lesson creates an interessement for the teenager to be taught in the same way as other "normal" school children, that is, to be normalised. This perception appeared to be an attractive emergent subjectivity, and the teenagers grasped the interaction as a school activity. Although this translation was possible, the materialities seemed to counteract it to some extent. Sandbacken is not a formal school; the art room is too small to be an ordinary classroom; the table was too big to be a desk; the teenagers were too few to be a class; and the teacher was not a teacher.

Investigation of the psychosocial situation

In interviews, the teenagers revealed that they knew that their actions were being interpreted and noted by staff members in order to investigate their behaviour (Severinsson, Nord, and Reimers 2015). Thus, colouring a heart with a black crayon and then destroying it may translate as an act leading to interpretations about the girl's psychosocial situation. It is possible that the action was noted in her records and discussed by the staff when devising a suitable treatment plan. Through the medical diagnostic lens, translations appear in which everything the teenager does and says is interpreted as a kind of performance of her psychosocial needs. The problematisation involves the staff's limited knowledge about the teenager's problems; and the solution is to investigate and get access to these problems and to appropriate treatment.

The materialities of the paper and crayon are then enrolled as test materials. The subjectivities in this translation are an investigation object (the teenager) with an investigator/detective (the staff member) interpreting her actions as a symptom of her psychosocial status. In this translation, the teenager emerges at the border between "normal" and being diagnosed or identified as in need of some kind of intervention. The interessement for the teenager is to be understood psychosocially, and the interessement for the care assistant is to understand.

Psychotherapy

The situation with the coloured and destroyed heart could also be a starting point for a conversation about the girl's psychological status and thus emerge as a psychotherapeutic session. The problematisation is then about the teenager's psychological trauma; and the solution is to talk about and work with the feelings. In this case, the teenager's actions are interpreted by the staff member as an aspect of her psychological (un)health, by the question: "Is this how you feel?" The girl destroying the paper and throwing it away opens up the possibility to understand her behaviour in this way.

If the network is viewed through this psychological lens, the paper and crayon are enrolled as a catalyst; that is, as a starting point for a therapeutic talk about feelings. In this translation, the teenager crosses the border of being an ordinary teenager and enters the subjectivity of a client or patient who is meeting a staff psychotherapist. The interessement for the teenager is having an opportunity to process emotions, and the interessement for the care assistant is containing difficult emotions.

Amusement

The art studio network could also be translated as a time-killer, allowing the teenager to do something (fun) for a while. The problematisation may then be about boredom, and the solution about having something to do. In contrast to the therapeutic framing above, in this translation, the teenager could have used and destroyed the material simply to tease and annoy the care assistant, as a way of passing the morning. Thus, the situation can be translated as innocent play that is not alarming or worrying. The material is then enrolled as garbage and the translation produces the subjectivities of an innocent teaser and an (also bored?) adult/parent. This translation's interessement makes it possible for the resident to pass as a bored teenager performing an activity that is similar to those occurring in many places in which "normal" teenagers spend their days.

Imprisonment

The staff member's question about how the girl feels is an important moment that may remove the risk of the art studio network developing into a detention home; that is, the risk of a prison translation. In a prison translation, the problematisation would be to a high degree about power and resistance. The girl would be enrolled as a prisoner or "problem child" throwing things and acting angry, and the staff member would be enrolled as a guard. The materials could be enrolled as a reward when the teenager is allowed to access the art studio, a test she obviously not would have passed.

Coercion and punishment might then be a threatening consequence. In the prison translation, discipline is lurking, imminent, embedded in the remote location; the impressive brick architecture of the building; and the staff's pseudo-pedagogical, pseudo-psychosocial and pseudo-psychotherapeutical knowledge. The prison network creates an interessement of the teenager not taking the situation any further, but either accommodating to it, as in this example, or putting up a fight in some way (resisting), as in other examples I witnessed.

This analysis reveals how different translations emerge from the network. The moment when the girl destroys the paper and raises her arm is crucial in all the examples. It is a moment at which many different trajectories may be embarked on. In retrospect, it is possible to look at the situation and ask questions that would never be asked in the flow of the network performance: What is she doing, and why? Is she disappointed in her perceived lack of ability to draw, is she demonstrating her psychological status or is her behaviour a starting point for an outburst or a fight? Is she aggressive? Thus, the mobilisation–that is, the future actions during which the network speaks with one voice–constitutes a shift away from other possible trajectories and translations, and gives way to certain relations in the network. All these different translations can shift quickly, and it is impossible for the actors to know what kind of translation is in play at what time. It is also possible to elaborate more than one translation at the same time. As the researcher, of course I also took part in these translations, reading the interaction through different discursive lenses. Such situations, with rapid shifts between different translations of the network, can be a way to avoid conflict and make it possible to continue activities. Here it is fruitful to discuss Pickering (1993) mangle concept, because the shifts can be interpreted as a way to handle resistance, albeit with a result that is not obviously accommodation. For example, if a conversation started to feel too personal or difficult, the teenager could shift to school mode by asking a question about the colouring. Similarly, the care assistant could use the investigation network to try to get to know the teenager, but then change to the amusement network and joke about something in order to avoid emerging conflicts and the disciplinary mode.

Employing the amusement translation or the school lesson translation is not as frightening or threatening as using the investigation translation or the psychotherapy translation. Both the teenagers and the staff members shift between these translations in everyday institutional life at Sandbacken. Thus, the enrolment of the materiality (the art room, walls, pencils, crayons, papers, table, chairs and little clay figures) also shifts, although the materiality still stabilises the translation. The temporally emergent conceptualisations in the network translations create an ambiguity that facilitates the continuation of interaction. Materiality is not creating resistance, as claimed by Pickering (1993), but is rather facilitating and enabling shifts by holding the situation together.

Producing new possibilities

Residential care homes for troubled teenagers are ambiguous, complex environments that are difficult to define and that offer multiple services at the same time. The use of the ANT concept of translation (Callon 1986) and diffractive methodology (Barad 2007) made it possible to capture this com-plexity and go beyond the more obvious discursive practices of discipline.

Because of the institutional ambiguity at Sandbacken as shown in its location architecture and furnishing, the art studio network offered many possible translations. It is possible to shift problematisations, interessements and enrolments and to produce knowledge and subjectivity going in different directions. By shifting between different translations, the teenage resident can remain a normal schoolchild having an art lesson, thus avoiding the subjectivity of a "problem child". The art studio gives teenagers the opportunity to perform the same activity with different outcomes. It also makes it possible to translate the art studio network in different ways and to shift between translations in rapid fluctuations. The materiality stabilises the network, but at the same time permits different readings about its emergent character. The material stabilisation of the various social fluctuations is enabled by shifts in the interpretation of the material aspects in an ambiguous environment. Minor materials such as crayons and paper, being used by people around a table in a small room with ambiguous connotations, contribute to the continual flux of flexibility and stabilisation.

The flow of different intentions and goals is constant, and the network possibilities can be said to shift between translations rather than being captured within the dialectic of accommodation and resistance, that is, the mangle (Pickering 1993). The openness provides an opportunity for several subjectivities to coexist, rather than positioning the teenager only as a person who is problematic and has to change. The staff can act upon one problematisation in one translation while the teenagers act in another. These shifts in translations prevent an open display of resistance and therefore diminish conflict. The mangle concept and the interplay between accommodation and resistance do not come into play in an observable way; instead, actors perform in parallel, simultaneous translations. The actors can use this ambiguity to rescue the network from breaking down in conflict; therefore, no one has to exhibit resistance or accommodation, and everyone can hold on to different subjectivities that fit a well-known or preferred version of translation. However, the rapid shifts between translations can be interpreted as a kind of resistance or accommodation in a very flexible or smooth kind of mangle.

The mobility and fluctuations in the translations of a residential care home present quite a paradox, because the staff members at Sandbacken often stated in interviews that the teenagers needed structure (Severinsson, Nord, and Reimers 2015). This analysis is an example of how a lack of "structure" and the translation of the network through different lenses make it possible to capture mobility and flow. In this example, the shifting translations can be viewed as an opportunity for staff members and teenagers to change between different interessements, or even to have different problematisations while remaining normal and accountable both as teenagers and as staff. The results of the analysis provide an example of the "paradoxical space" mentioned by Rose (1993) and Spandler (2009, 677) creating something other than mainstream thinking, which often includes very well-structured places for troubled teenagers. At first glance, the architecture of Sandbacken could make it an inappropriate building for the care of troubled teenagers, and its many layers of ambiguity could perhaps be described as an "unpromising configuration" (Philo and Pickstone 2009, 653). However, the architectural figurations–by their very vagueness–also produce unexpected strengths and possibilities for creating a network of non-stigmatised characters and avoiding the prison translation.

Notes

[1] A discourse is a certain way of thinking, talking and doing that determines what is possible and suitable to do. Foucault used the phrase 'discursive practices', because discourse is not given but is produced and reproduced through interaction. Discourse is materialised in the surroundings, and controls the actors while simultaneously being governed by the actors. In an early Foucauldian interpretation, people cannot think outside of existing discourses (Foucault 1970) however, Foucault later (1982) discussed how people can (try to) resist discourses.

CHAPTER THREE

STRATUM ARCHITECTURE:
AN ITERATED ARCHITECTURAL ASSEMBLAGE
OF CARE FOR THE VERY AGED

CATHARINA NORD

Travelling through time

Looking at the architectural plans for an almshouse constructed in 15th century Britain, it is surprising that several of the design components in that early architecture housing the aged and the infirm have been carried on into contemporary design models (cf. Godfrey 1955, and Regnier 2002). The model of rows of identical small bed-sitting rooms for residents along corridors or surrounding an open communal space is an architectural form that present-day facilities have inherited from their forerunners (Fig. 3.1). Existing assisted living facilities for seniors in need of 24-hour care are inscribed with a long tradition of care and housing for the aged, with roots in mediaeval monastic caring traditions in hospitals and old people's homes (Godfrey 1955). There are strong traits of community and fellowship inbuilt in these care homes. In the early days, religious life was a core constituent of common activities, which can be traced in spatial designs incorporating rooms for religious services. The ubiquitous chapel found in ancient hospitals and almshouses is not standard in contemporary facilities, but common living rooms and halls for shared activities, usually secular, but occasionally religious, remain. The dining hall featured in the almshouse plans reveals that residents took their meals together in mediaeval times (Godfrey 1955). This collective aspect of everyday life embedded in the architectural space has persisted into our time. Individuals who move in to assisted living are expected to take part in activities of various kinds together with fellow residents. This is an essential part of the care model and is regarded as best practice (Evans and Vallelly 2007).

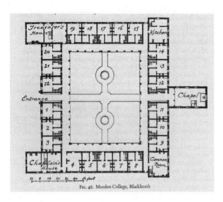
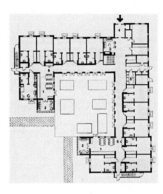

Fig. 3.1. There are striking design similarities between the plans of Morden College, opened around 1700 (left) and Postiljonen assisted living from 1994 (right). Both have common outdoor space surrounded by a corridor with small rooms for residents. Figure to the left from Godfrey, 1955, 64. Reprinted by permission from Mrs Arabella M. R. Hobson and family. Figure to the right from Regnier, 2002, 225. Reprinted and modified with permission from Wylie & Sons.

This paper will discuss why this architectural heritage has continued for centuries in light of the collective model of care associated with it. In the early 21st century, this model is increasingly challenged by alternative care practices in which the individual is strongly maintained as the centre of care. However, while assisted living care is subject to discursive changes, the architectural design of contemporary facilities is less prone to change in response to these new care ideas. The reasons for this inertia in the architectural design used in assisted living will be discussed on the basis of results from a qualitative study in two Swedish assisted living facilities. The analytic tools for this discussion are chosen from the Deleuzian-Guattarian toolbox, from which the concepts of *assemblage* and *stratum* provide the central theoretical structure of this story.

As a rule, assisted living in Sweden is provided in a small, quiet world of limited numbers and types of rooms in which very old, often immobile and fragile, residents are cared for by staff. Need for 24-hour care is a prerequisite to gain access to a place in assisted living. A visit outside meal times often reveals empty common spaces and closed doors behind which the residents rest, watch television, or read in solitude, occasionally calling for help from the staff. Visiting relatives irregularly add to the small number of people present. Although tranquillity reigns in these facilities and the routinely scheduled day usually has an undramatic course, I suggest that assisted living is a caring machine of great complexity; an assemblage of heterogeneous components (Deleuze and Guattari 2004). This is discernible, for instance, in the dilemmas that carers face each day while negotiating residents' competing individual needs. The fact that the residents are strangers to each other creates an ambiguous social life (Moore 1999). This is stimulating and vitalizing to some, but may be challenging to others, who try to avoid social encounters as much as possible by withdrawing to their rooms or detaching themselves from others in public spaces (Nord 2011a, Hauge and Heggen 2008, Andersson 2013).

Assemblage and stratum

The concept of assemblage has been used as an analytical tool for exploring buildings and architecture (Dovey 2013). An assemblage is characterized by movement and "becomings" in which associations between humans, material objects, and other components render possible the emergence of new understandings and functions. The interacting parts never merge into an inseparable whole. They keep a certain independence and can fall apart and enter new assemblages in new processes of becoming (DeLanda 2006). Thus, a building is a loose constellation of socio-spatial flows and fluid intersections, which permits an analytical focus on architecture as a set of processes and transformations separate from fixed forms and essentialism (Dovey 2013). In this type of analysis material aspects of architecture emerge as mouldable and dynamic. Buildings easily involve other actors in emergent processes by their ubiquitous presence. They are unavoidable and part of our everyday lives, but most often not present in our discursive awareness because "[t]hey become part of the unconscious background of our lives, rather than the focus" (Ballantyne and Smith 2012, 35).

Architectural research often starts with the house as a too-obvious object of investigation (Frichot 2005). Assisted living invites assemblage analysis by its defined architectural structure and its limited number of interacting components. Each assisted living building is limited in the scope of aspects that can be seen and grasped; it is tangible, present, and available for empirical research. However, the fact that it is a repeated model with horizontal and vertical connections in time and space makes every facility more than a separate building, but part of a spatiotemporal amalgamation that restrains the fluidity a building often has. The basic design has survived over centuries while producing similar design models at every period over an astoundingly long time. Assemblage has been used by others to endow an analytical structure to heterogeneous, mobile, and emergent processes (Marcus and Saka 2006), a method that is suitable for an analysis of assisted living as a whole. However, to understand the very strong inertia embedded in the architectural spaces of assisted living a special case of assemblage–the stratum–is also involved in this analysis[1].

The concept of *stratum* allows us to view the long repetition of architecture for care of the aged as an "imposed statistical order of connections and successions ('forms')" (Deleuze and Guattari 2004, 46). A stratum is a version of the assemblage with a higher degree of stability that gets its tenacity by double articulations in which it develops in two steps. The first articulation establishes a form from an aggregate of preliminary configurations (Deleuze and Guattari 2004). In the case of assisted living, the first articulation continued for centuries through a succession of architectural forms of caring institutions for the aged, materialized in an unbroken design chain, often under the auspices of the church but later integrated into the ambitions of the modern welfare state, moving from traditional to bureaucratic judicial authority (cf. DeLanda 2006, Åman 1976). The second articulation is the step in which the stratum is further predetermined and integrated, the stage that "establishes functional, compact, stable structures ('forms'), and constructs the molar compounds in which these structures are simultaneously actualized ('substances')" (Deleuze and Guattari 2004, 46). This second articulation happened in Sweden on 29 April 1993, when an addendum to the building regulations came into force, assigning assisted living its form through new design affordances (BFS 1993). Flats in assisted living in Sweden are legally on a par with ordinary housing and must follow the building regulations for other dwellings. However, the addendum deviates from the design requirements of ordinary housing in that it allows the flats in assisted living facilities to be of substandard size if they are juxtaposed with communal spaces, which are supposed to compensate for their reduced size (Nord 2013b). An architectural stratum was then confirmed and expressible, "actualized" both in the material world and in words (Deleuze and Guattari 2004). From that moment, assisted living could be talked about and understood as a certain form of architectural design in policies and practices of housing and care for older people. In fact, it became a standard model for future design, construction, and reconstruction (Nord 2013b). As a consequence, the architectural space is now more durable and inert than all other components of the assemblage of assisted living (people, furniture, food, animals, etc.). This model of architectural space breaks DeLanda's (2006) criterion of divisibility of the parts in an assemblage because the flats cannot be separated from the common areas without reverting them to the size required by the regulations for ordinary flats. If they are separated without being expanded to regulation size, they become illegal.

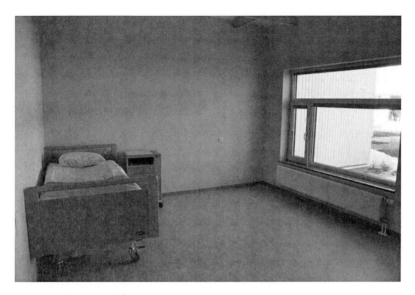

Fig. 3.2. Space for a restricted life in old age. Residents are invited to furnish their minimal rooms with a few of their own possessions. Photograph by Catharina Nord.

Assisted living was hereafter visible and "sayable". However, visibility in this context is not limited to all that can be seen, because the logic of the stratum makes certain phenomena appear "in the light", while others remain "covered up in darkness" (Deleuze 1988). In this case, discursive blindness relegated some ways of working to the dark corners of impossibility. The architectural stratum in assisted living is wedded to certain ways of working, implying a care model that is linked to this type of architectural form. Care for the very old and fragile is provided in a model focused on care for a collective, organized in routinized, repeated work tasks in a 24-hour cycle (Nord 2011a). This follows logically from the institutional architectural form and its legal framework, moulding a definition of ageing and care in this context. An architecture of this type contributes to collective and discursive blindness in which "irrelevant parts of the bodies, objects or concepts fade from view" (Ballantyne and Smith 2012, 20). Collective care is embedded in spatial instruments such as the legal transfer of square metres from private to public space, which implies a sacrifice on the part of the older resident in that every person renounces dimensions of privacy to gain the equivocal advantage of a life in public care. The minimal spatial provision of a bed-sitting room (Fig. 3.2 and 3.3) is more an accommodation of physical care work in a huge professional bed or bathroom than a decent space for a private everyday life, in all its diversities, in deep old age (Nord 2013a).

Assisted living is highly normative and disciplined, underpinned by a caring gaze, a collective organization, and a strong capacity to distribute people and things, similar to the institutions analysed and described by Foucault (1977). Furthermore, the addendum in the building regulations produces a normativity that reaches all the way to the work desk of the architect and blocks all possibilities of breaking up the regulated design and forming something entirely new (cf. Frichot 2005). A consequence is that assisted living in Sweden has never enjoyed the creative and liberating design processes that have transformed other disciplinary institutions discussed by Foucault, such as the school (cf. Dovey 2013).

The architectural components

There is nothing extraordinary about the architectural components of assisted living. Along with the residents' rooms it is assembled of mundane spaces with which we are familiar: corridors, kitchens, and shared dining/living rooms. These others can all normally be separated and continue to be corridors, kitchens, etc. when entering into new assemblages.

Many of the everyday spaces where we live and work presuppose the corridor's communicative and connecting capacities (Hurdley 2010). Office blocks, schools, shopping malls, hospitals, and even dwellings to some extent present the spatial logics of corridors-cum-other spaces. So, the corridor is conceivable in a number of spatial assemblages, even if a shift to another assemblage might change our understanding of and rationale for the corridor. While the corridor endows privacy and socio-spatial hierarchy in the family home by providing neutral passage to certain rooms (Evans 1978), in assisted living it is a tool for surveillance and the spatial distribution of collective living. Instead of the privacy the corridor renders possible in a dwelling, the corridor in assisted living endorses the Foucauldian gaze and the supervision of people in a number of disciplinary institutions such as prisons, hospitals, schools, and other establishments of correction (Foucault 1977). In most of these institutions, the corridor constitutes the architectural backbone and has been replicated in a variety of versions for similar purposes (Markus 1993). Thus, whereas the corridor is in certain assemblages a neutral means of communication, simply a space connecting other spaces (Hurdley 2010), in others it is a vehicle for power and surveillance (Foucault 1977, Markus 1993).

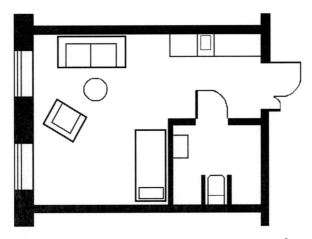

Fig. 3.3. General plan of a resident's flat in assisted living, about 30 m^2, with bed-sitting room, bathroom, and "kitchen"-wardrobe-entrance area. Drawing by Catharina Nord.

Similarly, a kitchen could be subjected to varied positioning. As a home space, it is linked to family relations, which changed during the 20th century in tandem with the redesign and redefinition of spaces in modern housing, including the kitchen (Putnam 1999). For instance, it is no longer clearly the woman's space it used to be (Saarikangas 2006). It is no longer associated with gendered subordination, which could even sever the kitchen from other home spaces and relegate it to memory or oblivion (Bordo, Klein, and Silverman 1998). The kitchen is a highly volatile and dynamic space, presenting a diversity of associations to things and people. Worldwide, it could be assembled of the most contrasting objects and technologies, such as African traditional cooking stoves (Jönsson 1991) or smart refrigerators and microwave ovens (Stander et al. 2012). It is not only the kitchen, but also the living room and dining room, that have been subjected to negotiations by modern living and changing family life, which has altered the human and non-human components of which they are assembled and offer links to other spaces. For instance, the bourgeois habit of a separate dining room has disappeared (Munro and Madigan 1999). The borders between dining room, living room, and kitchen have become blurred. While a living room is a public place where visitors are received and personal items are displayed "with the purpose of impression management" (Riggins 1994, 102), eating and leisure time activities may merge in front of the television (Munro and Madigan 1999) and the kitchen has become more presentable and less connected to cooking (Putnam 1999).

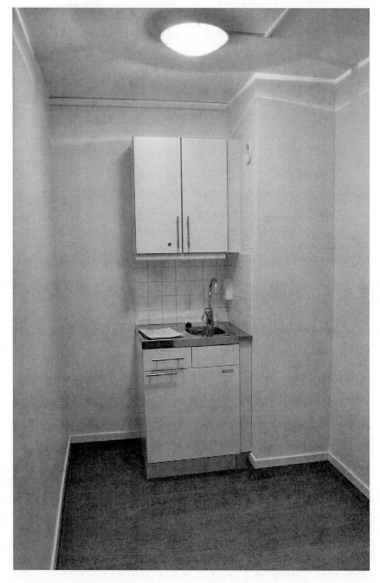

Figure 3.4. A symbolic kitchen in assisted living with no provision for cooking. Photograph by Catharina Nord.

Thus, a corridor, a kitchen, and a living/dining room can easily be transferred between a number of contexts and interact with various objects. However, in assisted living these common spaces (kitchen, living/dining rooms, and even corridors) are created from square metres removed from private space and reallocated, without which they could not exist. As a consequence, the residents' flats suffer from a lack of space, and this deprivation turns them into something similar to a student's dormitory room. Cooking is not possible. The "kitchen," or rather kitchenette, available is a legally prescribed, though mainly symbolic, metre of countertop. There are no hot plates provided and space for a coffeemaker and not much more. Electricity to the outlets may be disconnected, however, for security reasons if the resident shows signs of cognitive decline (Fig. 3.4).

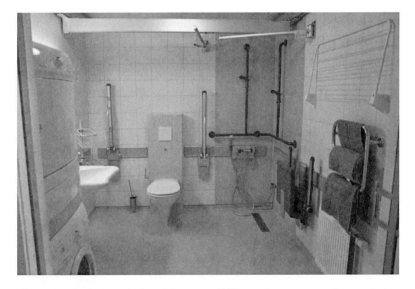

Figure 3.5. Bathroom designed for accessibility and to accommodate workplace regulations. Photograph by Catharina Nord.

The small flats provided for residents have extremely limited capacity for furnishing, so the residents may have to choose between a dining table and a sofa, because it is not possible to fit in both. The bathroom, designed for accessibility and to accommodate workplace requirements (Fig. 3.5), is oversized in such a small flat, comprising 10 m^2–approximately 25% to 30% of the total flat (Nord 2013a). A pertinent question is how many square metres can be removed from a flat before it can no longer still be called a flat? The minimal size of the flat forces the residents out in the public in accordance with the collective care model (Nord 2011b). In the dining room, the resident may find 15 strangers when entering for a meal. These people have all the same legitimate claims, since most of them (but not any staff who are also present) have contributed to the size of the room by foregoing some area from their flats. Hence, this jigsaw puzzle of legally defined bits and pieces, of which the dining room and kitchen now consist, cannot be separated into various components. This is why the architectural space is an extremely durable component of the assisted living assemblage, a stratum that is inert, unresponsive, stubborn, and immobile. However, this does not mean that there are no dynamics in the assisted living assemblage. There are other components which crave new connections and openings, searching for potential becomings.

The stratum and territorialization

Kim Dovey claims that *territorialization*, the dimension which stabilizes an assemblage, makes the concept the most relevant to architecture in the Deleuzian-Guattarian conceptual toolbox. Territory and space are associated with architecture in a number of ways. While territoriality is a stabilizing force, it is not just a state of immobility, but "creative rather than defensive, … establishing a zone of comfort and order, a sense of home that keeps chaos and difference at bay" (Dovey 2013, 135). The counter-process is *deterritorialization*, by which territories are challenged, transformed, and obliterated, and new associations are searched for and entered into (Deleuze and Guattari 2004). Deterritorialization can be highly disturbing, annoying, and awkward. It can also signal a craving for liberation.

The idea of individualized patient- or resident-centred care[2] emerged fairly recently as an alternative to anonymous collective care and is now a hallmark for the provision of good care to residents in assisted living (Yee et al. 1999). This has prepared the way for a new discourse of care in assisted living, with central goals such as resident autonomy, privacy, and dignity (Schwarz and Brent 1999). Resident-centred care deterritorializes assisted living by challenging its assumptions both in word and in practice. However, the ubiquitous architectural model of small resident rooms strung along a corridor and common rooms for meals and activities has proven to be a substantial obstacle to the introduction of other ways of providing care (Nord 2011b). The dominant care model with its architectural accomplice maintains the territorializing tensions in the assemblage of assisted living. The embedded stratum of the built environment in the assemblage of assisted living endows exceptional territorial abilities to defend the status quo and make it particularly resistant to deterritorialization. However, the two processes of territorialization and deterritorialization cannot be considered separately. They are rather subsumed; one is often the trigger of the other. The tensions in the assisted living assemblage are to a large extent created by the fact that there is an embedded stratum, an architectural model of great stability, which resists involvement in the dynamic processes of becomings by its dominance, inertia, and rigidity.

Words are means of territorialization by which an architectural assemblage is defended and upheld. They are deeply implicated in the production and use of buildings, and they might appear as buttresses against innovation and inventiveness (Markus and Cameron 2002). However, while being used to keep old-fashioned ideas stable, they might also, in the guise of new ideas, slip into minor chinks in the armour of the assemblage, like an almost imperceptible drip of water, and slowly undermine stable and solid edifices. "Here concepts link up with each other, support one another, coordinate their contours, articulate their respective problems, and belong to the same philosophy, even if they have different histories" (Deleuze and Guattari 1994, 18). The new concepts that have entered into the discourse of care in assisted living challenge the collective and community that are the core of traditional care and design. These concepts seek new associations which destabilize the assemblage (Deleuze and Guattari 1994). The contradictions between a number of binaries–private and public, individual and collective, surveillance and autonomy–are negotiated in architectural space with the consequence that a space of great ambiguity is created in which the continuity of the stratum is challenged. This is a battlefield where the connections between the actual and the potential may be revealed (Dovey 2013). New concepts articulate a new conceivable world looking for a spatial countenance (Deleuze and Guattari 1994). Processes of territorialization and deterritorialization occur until concepts merge and the spatial structure is destabilized. These processes cannot be analysed singly, they must be looked upon as an assemblage of mobile relations, subtle, tangible, and upsetting.

Deterritorializations of assisted living

The following examples illustrating deterritorialization in assisted living are drawn from interviews and observations collected in fieldwork during a qualitative study of the relationship between care work and architecture in two assisted living facilities in Sweden. A point of departure for this discussion is a perception of "care as tinkering" (Mol, Moser, and Pols 2010). This conceptualization views care as a practice in which tasks are done and redone until they are done as well as possible. It entails searching, trying, and testing various versions of similar actions. According to Mol and colleagues (2010), tinkering involves a diversity of materialities in caring in the form of technical equipment, grooming items such as toothbrushes, food, cutlery, animals, etc. Care as tinkering also includes negotiations about the spatial components of greater or lesser significance in the deterritorialization of assisted living.

Deterritorialization I: acknowledging space

One carer said in an interview:

> Each time I cross a threshold I meet a new person; then I have to reset myself before I enter and be another person–even though I am myself–I have to meet all people the same way by being different to them because they are different; they get the same ingredients, so to speak, but yet they get different parts of me depending on who they are. (Nord 2015, 16)

Caring as tinkering appears in this quote as an attempt to prepare for meeting a resident by adjusting the persona to create an individual encounter that will enhance the caring situation. In crossing an insignificant little architectural element, a threshold, her care approach deterritorializes the spatial fact that the resident flats are identical by acknowledging that the residents are individuals. It also indicates that she meets a number of residents during her work shift, perhaps repeating similar caring tasks that need to be adjusted to the individual. Moser (2010, 279) writes that:

> care approaches … are not made to reveal, transport and circulate truths about the situation on the ward, but are geared towards the persistent improvement of practices and care interactions.

Little is standard in the carer's work, few aspects are predetermined, and there is no such thing as an average resident. Or an average carer, for that matter. Each meeting is unique by the entanglements of a multitude of involvements. The carer cited thus prepares herself for the event in which her own and the resident's subjectivities coevolve as an effect of the caring encounter.

Architecture is a co-producer of its own and others' subjectivities in events where subjects come together in instantaneous and short-lived moments (Brott 2013a). This encounter yearns for a supple and malleable architectural space that embraces tinkering and contributes to the emergence of a good caring situation. The resident's private space is contested, ambiguous, and in flux, where qualities arise in the moment when they are performed (Nord 2011a). Disparities and the irreconcilable blend and appear in each other. Thus, private space might produce solitude or loneliness. Privacy is at stake in the moment that the carer–a complete stranger–works on the resident's most intimate body parts. Secrets a resident might want to conceal will be unveiled. Yet, the carer closes the door in a spatial deterritorialization, aiming for a private encounter with the resident. The gaze of others, both fellow residents and other carers, is excluded. Inside, there and then, is a private and intimate situation involving a resident and a carer to which no one else has access. However, how this develops is undetermined and unclear. The carer may have a certain task in mind on entering, perhaps morning dressing, assistance with cleaning, or reading a newspaper to the resident. However, the outcome of the event is uncertain until it happens. Morning dressing might end in a call to the doctor because the resident is not well, and the home space turns into a medical space. The newspaper might stay on the table if the resident is in a bad mood because she is convinced that she met her mother, dead for forty years, during the night before. The carer might try to get space and time in order, recalling the resident to the here and now. Then the agenda might change to comforting instead of reading, perhaps in the bed, holding hands, or hugging if the resident allows. Cleaning assistance might be delayed to listen to the resident generously share another story from a long life. Floor and surfaces might be neglected in favour of seeing and acknowledging the resident as an individual. Deterritorialization entails that space is occupied, even captured by life and care, to the extent that the borders between inhabitants and architecture are redefined and even obliterated. As Brott suggests: "[w]hen an architecture is truly inhabited, it is as if it begins to inhabit us" (Brott 2013b, 157).

Deterritorialization II: negotiating space

An architecturally distinct and spatially delimited dayroom and dining room in assisted living is a patchwork of square metres taken from the area of each individual flat. A seamless space with tables where residents dine together conceals this fact, and its existence depends on no resident claiming the right to the 10 to 15 square metres of public space that that person has conceded from the area of their private flat. However, deterritorialization may begin in more subtle ways, as in this straightforward utterance made by an 86-year-old female resident: "I have no interest whatsoever in socializing with anyone here." She put this intention into practice by spending all of her time together with her husband, mostly in their flat. Their public life included having their meals in solitude at a dining table at the end of the corridor outside their flat. The husband controlled their ambiguous privacy, snapping indignant eyes towards any co-resident who he suspected of approaching the table with the intention of using it. As a matter of fact, they deterritorialized common space by unwittingly claiming the right to the square metres of their flat they had sacrificed. Staff did not contest the couple's action nor did they interfere with this arrangement, even though they acknowledged that the privatization of public space was just barely acceptable. Most of the residents came to have their meals in the dining room anyway, at least during the first half of my fieldwork. However, suddenly a surprising rearrangement of the furniture in the dining room occurred. Two of the tables, which up to that point had been ordered in a row in the middle of the room where residents sat together at the meals, were scattered around the walls. Why this breaking up of the meals at a common table, including the pleasant afternoon coffee gathering with beautiful china, candles, napkins, and home-baked cakes–all the material-ities mobilized to facilitate the residents' participation? The simple answer was that some of the residents had refused to come to the dining room unless they got a table of their own. One could say that they had actually claimed the right to their individual public square metres, just as the couple did. This constituted a significant deterritorialization in the assisted living space. Although staff were embarrassed by the residents' claims, they took the requests seriously and rearranged the furniture, sacrificing the camaraderie of the afternoon coffees they had worked so hard to achieve. They refurnished the room (even visited storage and brought another extra table) so that people who wanted to sit alone could do that and those who enjoyed each other's company could still sit at a common table in the centre. Their efforts to improve the space for the residents were sincere and concerned. They deterritorialized the assemblage by destabilizing the collective model of care through strengthening both resident autonomy and privacy. However, the stratum interfered heavily with their negotiations in that the spatial demarcation of the dining room made it difficult to fulfil all requests and to organize functioning groups of people, since the space only accommodated a certain number of tables. Tinkering and trying by carers appeared in different guises. Some residents accepted sharing their table with one other person, and it was sometimes necessary to move residents to another table. One woman with severe dementia, for example, was moved to another table to protect her from the ladies with whom she was seated initially, who intimidated her because she had forgotten the conventional use of knife and fork. Unforeseen caring opportunities arose. A man who was deeply depressed and rarely left his bed was successfully tempted to come out by the promise of a table of his own in the dining room.

The limited space available in the dining room and in the residents' flats, which in most cases did not have space for a dining table, allowed the architectural space to resist deterritorialization. The residents were simply forced out to eat in public by the impractical furniture for meals in their flats. This practical side of life might have reinforced the carers' untiring efforts to persuade the residents to go and eat in the collective dining room and not in their private flat. Or was it the other way around? Space in the flat for a dining table is superfluous when one is expected to dine in public space. Territorialization is upheld by the visible and the utterable by certain forms of space and caring practices.

Deterritorialization III: a craving for space

The institutional preference for collective dining over residents dining alone in their flat was prominent in the case of a blind man's deterritorialization efforts to claim his right to privacy, autonomy, and perhaps even dignity. This man suffered from severe depression and wanted to lie in bed more or less permanently, which constituted a serious risk behaviour according to the medical assessment. A prolonged bedridden state exposes an already weak resident to the risk of pneumonia or other medical effects; as a consequence, this behaviour actually endangered the man´s life. The staff considered that his depressive state rendered him incapable of understanding the consequences of his choice of lying in bed all day. Biomedical ethics, in a case like this when a patient cannot make self-protective choices, require the staff to intervene by making proxy decisions to safeguard the person, sometimes against that person's will. The ethical dilemma involves how to help the patient to accept an unsolicited decision by the staff. Threats, punishment, and manipulation cannot be justified; the moral grey area concerns the use of encouragement and rewards to induce compliance in a patient (Beauchamp and Childress 2001). In this case, there were both discursive and spatial components embedded in the dilemma, restricting the options for both the resident and the staff. Avoiding pneumonia is fairly straightforward–the patient simply needs to sit up. The blind resident was not coerced into dining with his fellow residents, but the staff succeeded in persuading him to come and have lunch in the dining room, which he did, sitting at a table with three other men. The hidden agenda, of which the man was most probably not aware, was to make him sit up for as long as possible. After the meal finished, the staff left him at the table while all other residents returned to their flats, assisted by staff or on their own. Eventually only the man, one staff member, and I remained in the dining room. At this point, when the dining room had fallen silent, the man started asking to return to his room, which he could not do without assistance: "I want to go back to my room." When nothing happened, he repeated his demand, this time a little bit louder. The continued repeats of his request that followed grew in intensity and desperation until it was almost unbearable to listen to him: "I WANT TO GO BACK TO MY ROOM!" The man claimed his right to autonomy, privacy, and private space, totally against all biomedical advice, which is why staff had left him alone at a table in an almost empty dining room. His demand deterritorialized in a very substantial way the collective dining and common spaces while he claimed the right to a private home space by intangible means, voice, words, and utterances. He seemed to search for an answer to the problem that "home does not preexist: it was necessary to draw a circle around that uncertain and fragile centre, to organize a limited space" (Deleuze and Guattari 2004, 343). In the midst of an institutional care model in which collective care is the main objective, his true request for private home could not materialize because it was hidden in the shadow cast by medical discursive practices. Yet a solution to his problem was almost as simple as sitting up; a space was made for a dining table in his room. Thus, the staff's objective of having him sit up to prevent pneumonia intersected with his own desire for privacy.

Conclusions

Architectural space in assisted living is the backbone of routine work and reiterated interactions in a caring organization with roots far back in centuries past. Deleuze (1988) notes that Foucault gives precedence to statements over visibility in a stratum. So even if the architectural design stratum of assisted living operates as a strong protector of a collective caring model, in which any transformations are difficult to advance, contours of a new caring model emerge as a potentiality by that which is said. While the architectural model is the major territorializing factor furthering the resistance and continuity of the institution, whispers about individualized care appear as a vanguard, materializing into vague caring practices that may deterritorialize old truths and draft new possible associations that will eventually alter that which is visible.

Ongoing deterritorialization is fuelled in assisted living by the individuals who inhabit and staff the facility. So, despite the well-defined and homogeneous identity embedded in its self-protective stratum design, assisted living is destabilized by individuals' tinkering, negotiating with and around institutional routines, and seeking out care work that does not allow itself to be incorporated in the routinized narrative of the daily tasks. The three examples above illustrate that care as tinkering destabilizes binaries, categories, subjectivities, and iterative practices through risky and bold challenges. Residents' privacy, autonomy, and dignity are negotiated in refreshing deterritorializing processes in which architectural space is at stake.

Notes

<hr>

[1] DeLanda (2006) rejects the stratum concept in his elaboration of the assemblage theory, making the claim that they are the same concept. I prefer to see them as two closely related concepts with a strong family likeness, whose capacities are similar, though not identical, and of which stratum is the stronger, longer-lived version.

[2] Different types of concepts are used in different disciplines.

Commentary III

Sustaining the Webs of Life: An STS-Approach to Space, Materiality and Subjectivity in Care

Ingunn Moser

Spatial and material ordering in dementia care practice

During fieldwork in dementia care in a nursing home, I was struck by the complex and layered ordering of space and of time in daily life on the wards.[1] I will start with a few glimpses from my fieldwork:

On her daily rounds in the nursing home ward, Mrs. Hansen repeatedly expressed great relief and pleasure in meeting a familiar face, and hopefully also a friend, on her way. "What a surprise!", she would exclaim, "fancy we should meet here! What a coincidence! Puh - I am so pleased to meet you! Where are you going, what is your errand?"

As the conversation unfolded, it turned out that she was on her way to visit someone, family or friend. She would inquire about my whereabouts: how come we were on the same bus or ferry? Did I have origins or connections in the same area and community?

I was puzzled. How to think well about such incidents with persons with dementia? It would have been easy to reject it as phantasy, confusion or even hallucinations. But my job as an ethnographer was to be able to represent actions and interactions as rational on their own terms. So although we allegedly shared the same space, to my mind a typical institutional layout of a nursing home ward (long corridors with individual resident rooms, collective living rooms and the necessary facilities for bodily care work), there were obviously different spaces and different times being enacted at the same time. What was going on?

Mrs. Hansen was seated in a row along the wall, in a waiting mode, in a corridor or in a living room of a public kind. This was not very different from the typical situation in ferries transporting people across the fjords in Norway.

People would appear, either to enter and sit down with the crowd of passengers or to perform some work, and after a while people would leave again, probably to get off and get on with their different errands. There was no obvious shared purpose or connection among the people present, except the fact that they happened to find themselves in the same transitional situation.

Mrs. Hansen found herself to be among strangers. A stranger in an unfamiliar environment. No wonder she was struggling to make sense of where she was and how to move and behave herself acceptably. Garfinkel's (1967) and Sacks' (1992) renowned works on what it takes "doing being ordinary", i.e. passing as normal and competent, came to my mind. And if someone happened to behave themselves in a more private manner, for instance by lying down on the couch or putting their legs on the table or chair in front, this would usually call for reactions. This was interpreted as transgression: this was not home!

Mrs. Olsen, however, inhabited the collective space of the ward in a quite different way. She was a pastor's wife and had spent much of her life caring and catering for others people's needs. She was always alert and ready to assist laying the table, making tea or coffee or lending a helping hand. If it was late and dark and cold outside, she would fetch a blanket and a cushion and offer fellow residents or carers to stay over on the couch. To her, the ward was home, her fellow residents, guests, and the kitchen and living room arenas where she could take part in caring for others. As such, they offered Mrs. Olsen access to familiar and recognized subject positions. This also resonated with a more recent discourse the nursing home was trying to accommodate: reinventing the institution as home.

Even if the architectural and material premises of the nursing homes I visited as a researcher were older and shaped by other ideas than the most recent discourse in care policy, furnishing as well as practices and relations in the ward had been and were mobilized to make things more home-like. Resident rooms were redefined as private space and residents and their families were encouraged to bring private furniture, photos and other objects that could bring in a bit of home.

The objects that most often accompanied residents into the ward were photos. This also applied to Mrs. Hansen and Mrs. Pettersen. Mrs. Hansen and Mrs. Pettersen could often be spotted in the corridor waiting for their partners to visit. They would be watching out for a young handsome man, a fiancée or husband. Individually, they would invite the carers in to their rooms to show us their pictures and recall their stories. They would show photos of young elegant couples or young men in uniform. In otherwise "naked" institutional environments, these objects offered identification and contributed to maintain identities, memories and belonging. They reinserted one in connections of family, neighbourhoods, communities, work or natural environments–connections that were otherwise disarticulated and made absent. Along with historical photos decorating the corridors, these private photos continued to enact a life and a time past right in the middle of the here and now of the life on the ward. The only thing missing seemed to be the handsome young man. Why didn't he show up?

These situations and interactions in the ward made strong impressions. They taught me important lessons about the condition of dementia: how it is that this condition tends to make the world an utterly unfamiliar place in which people with dementia spend a lot of energy orienting themselves, figuring out connections, making sense and finding their way. And how it is that this takes place within and is shaped by specific material and spatial arrangements. Arrangements that may confuse, restrict or support the person with dementia in an estranged environment.

But the incidents also made me think about what we can learn from the condition and experience of dementia. Usually, dementia is conceived as something we need to learn *about* and understand in its deviance and progressive decoupling from the world, from "real life" and "real time". Hardly ever is dementia considered something we might learn *from*–for instance with regard to how it is we orient ourselves in time and in space in the first place. How it is we inhabit spaces. How it is we practice and negotiate spaces–and how it is that spatial and material conditions enable, but also restrict, the relations and expressions of life as well as of care.

What follows builds on a methodological impetus from ethno-methodological and ethnographic traditions in social science research that seeks to learn about the ordering of reality from within the practices and actors' own methods (Garfinkel 1967, Sacks 1992, Atkinson and Coffey 2001, Delamont 2004), and that accordingly assumes that actors, subjects and phenomena in the fields we study are able to bring both criticality and creativity to our disciplines.

Merits and limitations of an STS-approach

Depending on the context, I am a care researcher with a background in the academic field of science and technology studies (STS) or I am a second generation STS-researcher with an interest in health, care and their embodied and material conditions. Second generation STS-researchers have brought their STS tools and resources out from the scientific laboratory to study knowledge and knowledge practices in new and different locations, including care and daily life. As such, they have also transported and translated STS into new disciplinary and professional environments. Examples include health care, medicine and disability studies, but more recently also geography and architecture (Mol, Moser, and Pols 2010, Yaneva this volume).

In research in care, theoretical and analytical resources from the academic field of STS contribute to sensitize the analyses towards exploring, firstly, care as an embodied and in a wide sense material practice, relying upon and carried by an extensive network of relations. Secondly, STS interests and concerns focus on care as knowledge practice (Asdal, Brenna, and Moser 2007, Moser and Law 2007, Moser 2010a, 2011, Pols 2011).

From a STS point of view, it is empirically and theoretically intriguing to trace a multifarious knowledge practice such as care, involving an immense variety of tools, instruments, technologies and devices, from pills to toothbrushes, wheelchairs, hoists, cutlery, meals, bedrails, music, shields, curtains, locked doors and alarms. But also bodies, postures, positioning, voices, touch and eye contact. Not to forget the bodies of the carers as instrument of observation and registering. Care in formal and professional contexts also mobilizes methods, procedures, and research-based knowledge. Care mobilizes, tests and works on all kinds of elements and relations, in a tinkering and puzzle-solving mode. It tries out one thing at the time. It observes, registers, adjusts, and tries something else. It intricately qualifies each and every one of the elements in care interactions, but also the qualities of their interferences and interactions, in order to improve the condition of individual residents as well as of daily life on the ward (Moser 2010b)

In brief, then, STS-oriented analyses home in on and investigate the *practices* of health and care, in various locations, with various actors, networks and framing conditions, including those of material and institutional conditions. They are concerned with how these practices are ordered and shaped, but, crucially, also with what they aim and strive for, make possible and generate.

For instance, analyses of data from the dementia care ward demonstrate how an assumedly simple and routinized activity such as a meal situation was handled and organized, yes, with great care. As part of this, carers would also mobilize the spatial possibilities available to create distance or proximity, privacy or small collectives, for particular residents and for carefully chosen groups of residents. Sometimes someone would want to or have to be located at the margin of the collective. Sometimes residents were bothered, disliked or felt threatened by one another. Sometimes carers would add a shield, or find other means to create new spaces within the available space. In this way they would try–within the given premises - to cater for individual needs: for distance and privacy, for community and interaction. Carers would work to cater for and to protect the one and the many.

Sometimes carers would add something, and sometimes they subtracted something. In meal situations, cutlery could for instance be subtracted. If the extra complexity of knife and fork in a breakfast situation distracts you from the main task, namely that of eating, you are served ready-made sandwiches. If windows and glass doors turn out to be sources of stress, misunderstandings and scaring reflections, they are covered by curtains, flowers or the like to mute the stream of impression from the outside and to create a safe environment. If a bedrail may create the necessary safe space that enables rest, a bedrail may be added. In these and in multiple other ways, carers mobilize, make use of, work on, negotiate and creatively reinvent the given premises and conditions for care. And they do so in order to improve, to make things better: in care practice, but also in the individual condition of residents and the daily life situation on the ward. Care practice is inherently normative. In care it is not an option not to act. It is striving towards "goods", or qualities, that might contribute to improving the situation for those involved (Moser 2010b, Mol, Moser, and Pols 2010).

Translations of STS into new locations, practices and disciplines have contributed to a renewed concern with normativity. STS traces how normativities, qualities and strategies become embedded in materials and in arrangements, including spatial and architectural arrangements, that carry and shape practices. Further, the approach investigates how material and spatial arrangements contribute to normatively ordering and regulating social life, enabling certain practices, relations and positions while disabling others.

Based on this interest in the material dimensions and ordering of care in STS, one might expect a thriving discussion and body of work engaging with spatial and architectural conditions of care. But so far, this has not been the case. As in care research more generally, also STS research has defined its object of analysis and cut its networks in ways that tend to externalize actors like architecture and spatial conditions of care.[2] They tend to be treated as locations or arenas for action but are seldom made part of the object of scrutiny.

As for my own work, I have traced enactments of health care in and across different locations and practices. I have explored their different aims and values, actors, modes of knowing and resulting effects. I have had a specific interest in how various locations and practices become linked, or not, how they co-exist, and sometimes make part of networks and collaborate on concerns with health care. Empirically, I have investigated these concerns and questions in the fields of dementia care and in the rehabilitation and assistance offered people with disabilities in a Norwegian context.

This approach starts out from and stays put in daily life. It does not start in a discipline, laboratory or institution, assuming that their modes of knowing and understanding travel smoothly into other locations and shape practices and ways of thinking there. Instead, it traces if and how various actors, practices, forms of knowledge and locations become present, are mobilized and possibly contribute to enabling and regulating certain ways of living. I have for instance explored how new care policies and care schemes work out in practice. For this I have traced networks of relations that enable care and assistance from policy via service apparatuses to everyday life. I have investigated what kind of subjectivities are implied and made normative, how these become enabled and made possible in practice. Their bodily, material, technological and often also spatial conditions. The organization of service provision and the financial level of welfare underpinning them. Even the built environment and spatial conditions that contribute to enable (or disable) desired subject positions and gender identities (Moser 2016, 2005, 2017). But I have never started from the architectural and spatial conditions of various forms or locations of care to trace what kind of life, what kind of interactions, relations and subjectivities, they invite or restrict. Although my interest has been in care and its material conditions, spatial and architectural conditions have not been treated *symmetrically* in the analyses.

The promise of symmetry

So what is the promise of symmetry for analyses of spatial and material dimensions of care? What might a principle of symmetry bring in this context?

STS as an interdisciplinary academic field grew out of social and intellectual movements that formulated critiques of scientism and positivism, that is, the belief that science is a neutral, internally-driven supplier of neutral knowledge and a progressive force. On the basis of critical engagements with and analyses of the social relations, practices and contexts of science, existing theories of the relationship between science, technology and society became reformulated (Asdal, Brenna, and Moser 2007).

One of the creative centres in these engagements was the so-called *Edinburgh-school* with its Strong Programme and principle of symmetry. This demanded that all knowledge claims, regardless of success or failure, should be treated equally and explained sociologically. Rather than explaining scientific successes by referring to strictly epistemic and extra-social elements, and explaining rejected theories or failures by using social elements, the same sociological methods, conceptual tools and analyses should be used to explain both successes and failures -- regardless of how they were judged by posterity. Based on a particular reading of Thomas Kuhn's (1962) renowned philosophical insights on the development of scientific progress, they devised an empirical program for investigating and explaining the production of scientific knowledge as a social and cultural process.

This approach became radicalized in a further approach that aimed not only to overcome the division between science and technology on the one hand and society on the other, but also between human and non-human actors or agential capacities. The advocates of this approach, the so-called actor-network approach (ANT), argued that people, technologies, natural phenomena and other material objects can all be components in materially heterogeneous actor-networks and take on the role of actors.

Starting from semiotic traditions and their insights into how things come into existence as a result of the set of relations of which they are part, ANT expanded this to apply also to other, material kinds of entities. It is not only meaning that is relational, according to ANT: natural science's truths, technology's (or architecture's) material dimensions, and sociology's actors and subjects exist only as the effect of the set of relations they constitute. The basis of this *material semiotic* approach is that objects and subjects, facts and artefacts, material and social conditions, and social actors and practices, are equally made and sustained in and by means of ongoing relations (Law 2004). But what is more: they emerge together, in the same processes. A care practice necessarily has spatial dimensions and involves a spatial practice and production. An architectural process aiming to literally making space for care, necessarily envisages care relations and devises care practices. The spatial and material on the one hand and the social on the other emerge, and are attributed and ascribed characteristics and qualities, from their network of relations. They are "co-produced" (Asdal, Brenna, and Moser 2007).

Interestingly, this is also where STS and the non-representational approaches supporting the contributions to this volume meet: both approaches treat reality neither as a given nor as socially constructed. What they share is an analytical interest in what one might call "worlds-in-the-making". Worlds-in-the-making are studied as continually assembled and arranged, rather than given in an order of things, and as simultaneously discursive, social and material. They draw on many common resources. For instance, they adopt the thesis of "discourse" as a "strategy in materials" from Michel Foucault (1981). Accordingly, knowledge and discourse are understood to be performative, generative and literally mattering.

However, and as this volume also argues, it is well established that architecture is material culture and contributes to material ordering. What STS and non-representational approaches add is that not even architectural ordering is given or unambiguous. As several chapters in this volume demonstrate and the above excerpts from fieldwork suggest, the capacities of architectures and material ordering to discipline and restrict (as well as to enable and empower) are limited. Following Law (1994), order is better treated as a verb, as order*ing*, than as a noun. It is iterative, precarious and never finished. It is nonetheless normative and performing a kind of "ontological politics" (Mol 1999) in the sense that any ordering endeavour articulates and contributes to specific worlds-in-the making, and dis-articulates other possibilities (Law 2004).

Practices, then, including spatial practices, tend to escape their material as well as discursive regulation and conditions. Material and spatial arrangements become enacted, and endowed with agential capacities, but they also become negotiated and reinvented. New ideas and discourses tend to interfere with what is already there. Different discourses, strategies and ordering modes usually co-exist and also interfere with one another. This explains both the complexity and the openness in situations, in practice. In line with this, space is perhaps better understood as an effect or an achievement of material practice (Mol and Law 1994), and as such intertwined with practice, rather than simply conditioning, carrying or containing it. Symmetry, in this context, implies that these concerns with space and with (care)practice are equally attended to and articulated in and as one process.

This book certainly contributes to the drafting of such a symmetric approach. This volume is therefore highly appreciated and welcome. It includes a fine collection of contributions that deal empirically and theoretically with the performativity of architectural space and regulation, as well as with spatial negotiations and spatial creativity in care practices and care institutions. As such they make substantial contributions to STS.

The other way around, the concerns, sensibilities, tools and resources of an STS-approach have much to offer studies of architectural and spatial processes, in care, institutions and beyond. The material semiotic approach, which traces realities as made and sustained in and by means of ongoing relations, lies at the heart of this. It includes the individual care relations, the social relations and networks they are embedded in, in families and communities as well as in professional care organizations, and their embodied, material and spatial premises. It treats all these human, social and material realities as emerging in one process, one web of relations, and it offers the tools needed for tracing the conditions for these webs of life.

Care as sustaining the webs of life

In previous work, I have demonstrated that different care practices act upon and enact dementia in different ways–ways that shape distinct ways of living and dying with dementia, and create and distribute possibilities differently

(Moser 2011). I argued, and argue again, that a relational approach to life and dementia offers wider possibilities for action in terms of care as well as patient agency and subjectivity, than more somaticizing practices. As the introductory excerpts from fieldwork showed, and I expand on in the following paragraph, this also applies to architectural and spatial dimensions.

With Mrs. Olsen, carers found ways of engaging her in daily life practices, particularly situations involving meals, around the coffee table or evenings with television news. These little tasks and initiatives gave access to positions in interactions where she became acknowledged as a competent person: a generous host, a good housewife, a caring neighbour or friend. She got access to a whole repertoire of positions that were familiar, that built connections to her previous life, offered identification and worked to sustain her subjectivity.

For others, including Mr. Nilsen, a strong and energetic man with a history as football player and referee, but also a wildlife and nature lover, the sheltered garden offered possibilities for participation and meaningful activity. In addition to flowers and plants offering sensual pleasures and memories, and paths that allowed residents to go for walks in a safe environment, the garden also housed a shed with some tools and a heap of earth. This became Mr. Nilsen's precincts. Here he could shovel earth, work undisturbed and contribute to a common good: the garden.

The nursing home had also refurbished some office areas and established its own traditional hair salon. Here a local hair dresser invited customers from the nursing home a few days a week. To behave and comport oneself properly and competently in a hair salon, i.e. be seated in a waiting area, waiting one's turn, having a look in a newspaper or a magazine, small talking or just letting the hairdresser get on with her work, seemed to be an easy social task that also offered residents valued positions beyond those of "patient", "dependent" and the one in need of care and assistance. Along with the garden, the hair salon and the practices it brought in, contributed to expand the repertoire of positions, and equalize the relations between positions, in care offered in the nursing home. They helped build more symmetric relations. Agency became somewhat more symmetrically distributed. Carers were not the only active agents and residents not only passive care recipients, fixed in positions of dependency.

This relational approach to dementia in care practice works to engage and invite residents into positions and interactions where they can be recognized and acknowledged as competent actors and subjects; experience identification and connection; and share in meaningful activities, exchanges or relations. In this relational mode of ordering, then, life *is* being related, or being in relation. Relations are of course human, and imply experiencing connection and belonging. But there is more to it. These relations are also embodied. They are for instance sensual and tactile. Then there is the social dimension, with the mutual recognition and contribution that make a collective and carry its practices. But the relations that make life are also material and spatial. They involve a heap of earth, a shovel and a shed in a garden. The coffee, the porcelain, a cushion and a blanket. A hairdryer and hair salon. These material elements also go into the web of relations that make and sustain us as subjects and persons.

The insight into the relational interdependence of people as caring subjects, is a central motive and force also in care ethics (Barnes 2012, Barnes et al. 2015). According to Tronto (1993), people exist in and through caring relations with others. This is a classical formulation of care ethics. But Tronto also takes us beyond such a dyadic approach. According to her, care is constitutive of human being as well as of social and public life. And, what is more, care is an "activity that includes everything that we do to maintain, continue, and repair our "world" so that we can live in it as well as possible. That world includes our bodies, our selves, and our environment, all of which we seek to interweave in a complex, life-sustaining web" (Tronto 1993, 103).

So care is concerned with the life-sustaining relations that carry life and build worlds. Webs of relations that include the spatial and material. In light of this, it also makes sense to speak of a caring architecture. What I have tried to show and argue here, is that an STS-approach offers resources for tracing the threads and exploring the textures and materials of such webs of life, including the "how", the processes of interweaving, empirically.

Notes

[1] The empirical data this article draws on were collected as part of a research project on Alzheimer's disease in science, politics and everyday care practices. The fieldwork took place in sheltered units for people with dementia in two different nursing homes in Norway in 2006-2007. It was based on participant observation, interviews and informal conversations, and document analysis. The project was approved by the regional research ethics committees and NSD. Data have been altered in order to protect the anonymity of patients and carers.

[2] There are notable exceptions, including Mol and Law (1994), Schillmeier and Domenech (2010), and Pols (2016).

CHAPTER FOUR

"ENGINEERING" AFFECTIVE ATMOSPHERES AND THE ROLE OF AESTHETICS IN THE ASYLUM

KIM ROSS

Introduction

> The treatment of the insane is conducted not only in, but by, the asylum. (Fairless 1861, 7; original emphasis)

In sharp contrast to the bedlam of the eighteenth and early-nineteenth century madhouse, the asylum, as a result of shifts in opinion regarding the treatment of the insane and the associated mid-century reforms, was a highly designed and engineered space, viewed as a crucial device in treating and managing the insane. Although buildings had long been used to constrain and segregate the mad, by the nineteenth century it was recognised that they could be designed and manipulated in such a way so as to classify populations, enabling more tailored management and treatment, and could also be engineered to produce certain behaviours within the population (see e.g. Tomes 1994, Topp, Moran, and Andrews 2007) Consequently, they were viewed as a powerful tool, central to controlling and producing docile patients within the carefully planned spaces.

This recognition that asylums, as multifaceted spaces, were engineered to embody a number of responses in the inhabitants through the (often subtle) manipulation of environments is central to this chapter. By the second half of the nineteenth century, asylums were designed to control, to restore *and* to calm through careful planning and management. The internal and external spaces were continually evolved and transformed, not simply as a coping mechanism in the face of ever-increasing patient numbers, but also predominantly with the fundamental aim of returning "the mad" to reason in curable cases or creating a home-like, "hospice" environment for non-curable patients (Ross, 2014).

The chapter will begin by more formally positioning the theoretical underpinnings before moving to elaborate the conceptual material. Specifically, attention will firstly concentrate on explanations of *affect* and *atmosphere* in non- and more-than- representational literatures before moving to examine how these theories have been applied in studies of architectural geographies. These concepts will be used as the foundation for understanding the "engineering" of affective atmospheres into architectural spaces. Merging this with a Foucauldian understanding of the power relations in asylums, it will become clearer how those in positions of authority were able to use affective techniques and engineering as a mechanism to control how bodies acted in response to their (socially and politically constructed) environments.

The chapter will then move to explore the difficulties of employing non-representational theories in historical inquiries where the main source of evidence is words, which are, by admission, representational. The empirical evidence will offer ways in which this challenge can be navigated, namely through the recognition that the focus will be on uncovering the *potential* affective powers within asylum spaces. Contrary to Pile's assertion that affects "cannot be grasped, made known or represented" (Pile 2010, 9), it is argued that those in positions of authority (in this instance Commissioners, politicians, superintendents and architects) *do* have the necessary capacity consciously to manipulate, engineer and control affectual spaces, in order to influence the behavioural and emotional responses of people inhabiting those spaces. Thus, although the patient voice is "missing" within the archive, it is possible, as will be explored below, to uncover the *potential* of affect, or the desire to create affective spaces, and the *will* of the powerful to create and manipulate such spaces. Through historical records, the discussions, actions and motivations of contemporary actors responsible for the construction of asylums can be observed, uncovering their *will* to manipulate space, bodies and behaviour, yet still recognising that this will cannot always be traced through to exposing the emotional responses to such engineered affects on the ground, thus remaining *potential*.

Geographies, affect and non-representational theory

Recently, there has been a turn in geography and across the social sciences towards the study of affect (see Pile 2010, Thien 2005, Thrift 2004). This expanding "affective turn" has occurred as a response to an apparent absence of emotions within academic research and practice; an attempt to comprehend how the world is negotiated by feelings, forces and drives. This takes "geographical knowledges ... beyond their more usual visual, textual and linguistic domains", towards understanding emotions "as ways of knowing, being and doing in the broadest sense" (Anderson and Smith 2001, 8). The study of affect is connected to emotions, with ontological distinctions commonly drawn between the two terms. The latter refers to the emotions that individual humans feel, perceiving in a perhaps corporeally bio-physical sense (a "sinking feeling", a "light head") but certainly as an altered state-of-being in the world (happy, sad, elated, depressed, angry, resigned etc.), which arguably becomes cognitive and can usually be self-consciously identified, named and talked about (even if the words inadequately represent the sensations and perceptions). More complexly, affect denotes the prior force that impels the emotions or, more generally, impels a response in an "other" thing; usually conceived of a human having an emotional response, but it could be an animal instinctively running away or even a paper turning yellow (Lorimer 2008, Wetherell 2012), a response, according to Pile (2010), regarded as non/pre-cognitive on the part of the responding thing. Affect is the "material" connection–that which moves, travels, resonates, chimes across from one "thing" or body to "another", travelling between entities or bodies–which can encompass "things, people, ideas, sensations, relations, activities, ambitions, institutions, and any other number of other things, including other affects" (Sedgwick 2003, 19). Thus, affect can be defined as a material "force" impelling changes, responses, re-actions and emotions, and is consequently concerned not with the singular body, but with the relations between bodies (Pile 2010).

The definitions of, and connections between, affect and emotion have been outlined and contested by a number of geographers, for example Pile (2010), who argues that there are important conceptual differences which should be respected, while Bondi and Davidson (2011, 595) reply: "emotions, feelings and affects present us with messy matters to work with; they are tough to 'see', hard to hold, even trickier to 'write up'. But this is the nature of the beasts". Recognising these disagreements, for this chapter the crucial point is the appreciation that these affects/emotions can be consciously and politically manipulated (Sharp 2009), particularly by those in positions of power, through the specific engineering of bodies, space and atmospheres, which can be produced in such a way so as to create certain performances, or the potential for a desired performance, within those spaces: "the presumption that the powerful can manipulate the non-cognitive" (Pile 2010, 14).

New research on affect within the social sciences approaches the term from different directions. For many, their interest is topic-based, "infusing social analysis with what could be called psychosocial 'texture'" (Wetherell 2012, 2) which results in a focus on embodiment; how people are moved, what attracts them, feelings and memories. For others, the affective turn is more extreme, "a more extensive ontological and epistemological upheaval, marking a moment of paradigm change" (Wetherell 2012, 2-3). For Pile (2010), affect is indeed non/pre-cognitive, interpersonal (or even transpersonal) and inexpressible (thus non-representational), while Anderson (2006, 735) defines it as "a transpersonal *capacity* which a body has to be affected (through an affection) and to affect (as the result of modifications)". The affective turn in geographical research predominantly lies within this theoretical shift, following the philosophies of, among others, Spinoza, Deleuze and Massumi (or as Pile (2010, 8) summarises "Brian Massumi's reading of Gilles Deleuze's reading of Spinoza's account of affect"). This marks a significant turn away from critical theory based on discourse and disembodied language and text, to "more vitalist, 'post human' and process-based perspectives" (Wetherell 2012, 3). Geographies of affect, according to Thien (2005), are interested in researching this "how" of affect, with focus on the *potential* of the virtual, following Massumi, who argues that "affects are virtual synesthetic perspectives anchored in (functionally limited by) the actually existing, particular things that embody them" (Massumi 2002, 35-36). Thrift in particular has written considerably on the theory of affect, perhaps most noticeably his 2004 essay on the spatial politics of affect. Of crucial relevance to this chapter, he believes affect to be:

> more and more likely to be *actively engineered* with the result that it is becoming something more akin to the networks of pipes and cables that are of such importance in providing the basic mechanics and root textures of urban life ... a set of constantly performing relays and junctions that are laying down all manner of new emotional histories and geographies. (Thrift 2004, 58 emphasis added)

Approaching studies with an awareness of affect allows researchers to "trace the insidious ways through which power works on and produces bodies" (Dawney 2011, 600), as well as having great importance in allowing the world to be comprehended as externalities, where individuals, concepts and materialities develop as a result of material practices, objects, institutions and so on. In other words, "different sets of things, their configuration, their assemblage and spacing; their energy, have different capacities to do different things" (Bissell 2010, 83), with Toila-Kelly (2006, 2) arguing that it is essential to recognise the "power geometry" of these capacities to affect or be affected. Thus, contrary to Pile's assertion that affects "cannot be grasped, made known or represented" (2010, 9), it is argued that those in positions of authority (in this instance Commissioners, politicians, superintendents and architects) *do* have the necessary capacity consciously to manipulate, engineer and control affectual spaces, in order to influence the behavioural and emotional responses of people inhabiting those spaces.

Affect, atmosphere and architecture

Anderson believes that the notion of affect is best understood as "the transpersonal or prepersonal intensities that emerge as bodies affect one another" (Anderson 2009, 78), and that in everyday speech this notion is summed up by the term "atmosphere". He argues that this term navigates differences between peoples, things and spaces; therefore, for example, "it is possible to talk of: a morning atmosphere, the atmosphere of a room before a meeting, the atmosphere of a city" (Anderson 2009, Pile 2010) and so on. Indeed, he ponders that perhaps atmospheres envelope all things, with everything being able to be described as atmospheric.

The concept of atmosphere is interpreted slightly differently by Böhme, who focuses on the spatialities of atmospheres, relating more to the material roots of the word: "*atmos* to indicate a tendency for qualities of feeling to fill spaces like a gas, and *sphere* to indicate a particular form of spatial organization based on the circle" (Anderson 2009, 80). By this definition, it can be understood how atmosphere can surround people, things and environments:

> Thus one speaks of the serene atmosphere of a spring morning or the homely atmosphere of a garden. On entering a room one can feel oneself enveloped by a friendly atmosphere or caught up in a tense atmosphere. (Böhme 1993, 113-114)

The characteristic spatial form of an atmosphere is therefore dispersion within a sphere, having the ability both to envelope and/or to radiate from, an individual or object, including buildings. Consequently, as put forward by Deleuze and Guattari and highlighted by Anderson (2009), multiple types of bodies, which affect each other on a daily basis, produce various atmospheres and, crucially for this chapter, these atmospheres can be potentially shaped:

> Practices as diverse as interior design, interrogation, landscape gardening, architecture, and set design all aim to know how atmospheres are circumvented and circulate. By creating and arranging light, sounds, symbols, texts and much more, atmospheres are 'enhanced', 'transformed', 'intensified', 'shaped', and otherwise intervened on. (Anderson 2009, 80)

It becomes clearer, then, that it is possible to *engineer* "affective atmospheres" through attention to, among other things: light, colour, sound, shape, temperature, arrangement, texture, objects and people, with many of these measures belonging to an architectural sphere. Different feelings and emotions are suggested and enabled by, for example, designing an apartment to have a specific outlook, arranging the layout of a room or choosing specific aesthetic objects to create a certain feeling within a space.

Bodies can be affected in an almost unlimited number of ways (Kraftl and Adey 2008), but engineering spaces and atmospheres through architectural, landscape and interior design is a way of stabilising and controlling affect "to generate the possibility of precircumscribed situations, and to engender certain forms of practice" (Kraftl and Adey 2008, 228). One of these aspects that embraces the engineering of affect is therapeutic space, which can be defined as "spaces emergent through the enactment of practices that explicitly attempt to facilitate a kind of transformation in awareness, thinking, feeling and relating" (McCormack 2003, 491), with a specific sense of engineering therapeutic atmospheres. Indeed, as Kraftl and Adey state, "for architects and their buildings to be taken seriously, buildings must be imbued with the power to make a difference to their inhabitants" (Kraftl and Adey 2008, 213); for example, to feel "home-like" even if they are not a home (Kraftl 2010).

Creating affective atmospheres as a political decision

Kraftl and Adey's research considers this manipulation and engineering of architectural space, looking at both the creation and limitation of affect within certain buildings. Their emphasis goes beyond generic kinds of architectural affect (such as "homeliness", "comfort", or "peacefulness"), instead focusing "on the definite, desired affects that–through design– should be properties of the buildings, if the designs are effective" (Kraftl and Adey 2008, 215). They recognise the performative connection between a building and an individual: architectural designs are "imbued with styles of bodily doing, because of the push that the particular relationship between a body and that building could bring about: an affect" (Kraftl and Adey 2008, 217). Following Thrift, they recognise that designing particular affects into, and out of, a building is a "political" decision and, "though affective response can clearly never be guaranteed, the fact is that this is no longer a random process either. It is a form of landscape engineering that is gradually pulling itself into existence, producing new forms of power as it goes" (Thrift 2004, 68). By this reckoning, individuals' behaviour and emotions can be controlled by the manipulation of affective spaces within particular institutions. Yet, Kraftl and Adey (2008, 219) caution that, "there is not (and could never be) a neat or complete correspondence between the design of affect and its experience; the creation, evocation, and experience of affect is just not like that", as it is never certain how an individual will respond. As a result, as alluded to above, spaces can only ever be engineered and designed to be *potentially* affective: there will always be "gaps" between the engineers' interior and how a building's dwellers experience, receive and respond to the affective atmospheres being engineered. Kraftl and Adey (2008, 228) conclude by opening up the invitation for more studies to focus on the non-representational aspects of the built form:

> There is a need to explore the importance of a variety of architectural designs, forms, and inhabitations that try to embrace, manipulate, entrain, channel, push, pull, and create different capacities and collectivities for dwelling, and for affect production.

It must be recognised, therefore, that buildings, in their many forms, play a significant part in the daily lives of the majority of individuals: "they embody the literal act of place-making" (Kraftl 2010, 403). There are of course embedded power relations within, and attached to, these buildings. This claim follows Lefebvre, who explores the notion that "space is not merely produced for simple consumption, but [rather] spaces can be adapted, manipulated, appropriated, and produced by a range of individuals" (Llewellyn 2004, 229). Developing this point further, Lees, like Kraftl and Adey, believes that not enough is said by geographers on the non-representational and affective aspects of architecture, and that more attention should be directed towards the "embodied engagement with the lived building" (Lees 2001, 52), since the inhabitation of the building is just as important as its physical form and architectural type. Practical engagement with the "situated and everyday practices through which built environments are used" (Lees 2001, 56) is essential in understanding the occupancy of the specific spaces and places of a building. This leads to considering the individual consumption of architecture, asking questions about what the architecture *does* to its inhabitants (or what it is *trying* to do) rather than what it *means,* as well as questions about how people "dwell" in buildings, streets and other structures:

> No longer just a passive stage for the rehearsal and re-presentation of predetermined social scripts, space becomes alive and integral, inextricably connected to and mutually constitutive of the meanings and cultural politics being worked out within it. (Lees 2001, 72)

This orientation becomes difficult from an historical perspective, as understanding what a building was designed to *do* to its inhabitants in the past, through the engineering of affective atmospheres as outlined above, requires an interpretation of the available archive material. Often allowing no proper recovery of the actual everyday practices of individuals within the spaces concerned, the archive can be used to understand how past architects and planners have calculated and designed affective *blueprints*, incorporating the means *potentially* to affect the building's inhabitants (a further illustration that affects are always becoming and emergent). Drawing from Jacobs' work on "big things" concerning the *making* of buildings, archival analysis can, to some extent, uncover "the ways in which certain architectural forms come to be in certain places" (Jacobs 2006, 3), and, extending this idea, how they were designed to be affective. Through an examination of the archival documents, the building no longer appears as a final "fixed" entity, but rather there is scope to "interrogate the conjoined technologies (pipes, bricks, cabling), practices (construction, inhabitation, even demolition) and regulations (laws, building codes, health and safety legislations) that ensure they stand up over time" (Kraftl 2010, 407-408). An insight into the production and creation of affect within architectural spaces can, then, be read from archival sources. As will become evident in the examples to follow, affectual language, or *potential* affectual language, can be gleaned from the archive, giving an insight into architectural decisions and how individuals were manipulated to react (emotionally and physically) in desired ways when they were brought together in certain designed spaces. Although unable, in many instances, to uncover the bodily and emotional responses to the affective atmospheres and power relations created, reconstructing the *blueprint* and the desired *potential* outcome written in historical documents becomes a useful tool in constructing the methods of power deployed in an historical context.

Engineering affective "asylum" spaces

For the most part, nineteenth-century Commissioners in Lunacy actively promoted the spatial separation of the insane from society in purpose-built asylums. This process of exclusion was motivated by a desire to place particular people in perceived therapeutic environments, but always with an undercurrent of social control and custody, as, it should be recognised, therapeutic environments, supposedly designed to create individuals capable of re-taking their place in society as "docile bodies", were of course also a form of ("soft") social control (Foucault 2006): persuading the insane to "perform" sanity. Central to this ambition was the crafting of physical spaces for rest, relaxation and recreation within the asylums. Moreover, there was at bottom a profoundly "environmentalist" conception, with the Scottish Commissioners in Lunacy (SCL) relying on the affective qualities of the place in which the mad person was to be consigned. Indeed, as the nineteenth century progressed there was an increased understanding that "the condition of the insane is modified by the nature of their accommodation" (Scottish Commissioners in Lunacy (SCL) 1873, viii), resulting in still more attention to the external and internal aesthetics of the asylum. These views were embedded within the wider movement of reducing restrictions on liberty, as it was advocated that more could always be done to "secure the contentment of the patients so that they might the more readily conform to what was required of them" (SCL 1881, xliii).

It was thought that attention to micro-spatial arrangements was useful, "not merely by conferring temporary ease or pleasure, but also, and chiefly, by raising the general *mental tone* of the patients, and making them more amenable to treatment" (SCL 1862, lxxx, emphasis added). Here reference to the "tone" of people and place precisely suggests a concern for creating affective "atmospheres" with, over the study period, increasing attention paid to developing a "home-like" ambiance and a "comfortable domestic appearance" (SCL 1864, li) within the asylum. It was recognised of these efforts that:

> They may not, it is true, directly affect the health of the patients, but they tell directly on their comfort; and if it be the case that nine-tenths of asylum inmates are incurable, it is evident that attention to these details must be of as much practical importance to the bulk of the patients as medical supervision in its restricted sense. (SCL 1870, xlvii)

Crucially, the sense conveyed in this quote and those that follow was that, due to the accumulation of chronic patients, these developments were less about cure–as in older/original claims about "moral architecture"–and more about general orderliness through the creation of spaces capable of soft control.

Architecture

Architectural design and spatial organisation, which includes the construction and reorganisation of space at various scales, is an important means in creating affective atmospheres (Kraftl and Adey 2008). This was clearly evident in nineteenth-century asylums, which were often impressive, large scale establishment of considerable size and extent. The Inverness Asylum, for example, served the whole Highland region, including the Western Isles. In theory the patients were meant to feel secure and comfortable in these surroundings but it must have been difficult for people from small crofting communities to feel at home in this bewilderingly large, rather formal institution. To combat this issue, it was suggested in 1873 by the Commissioners that, in order to achieve tranquillity in the larger asylums, each ward should be arranged as if it were "a small independent establishment" (SCL 1873, lii).

The district boards continually sought to modify the physical structure of the asylum buildings, again to produce the most a/effective arrangement for the treatment and management of the patients. In 1878, it was reported that the Perth Asylum had "undergone extensive structural changes" which not only considerably increased the accommodation, but also involved "the removal of many grave structural defects in the old asylum building" (SCL 1878, xlviii). Along with updates to the fittings and furniture, the changes placed the asylum "in harmony with the most advanced views of treatment, and render the house a cheerful and comfortable place of residence" (SCL 1878, xlviii). In a similar vein, the Stirling Asylum was said to have improved its accommodation through simplifying the arrangements of the interior of the building; and, although the report did not give detail as to exactly what was altered, it did state that as a result "its efficient management has been greatly facilitated" and that "much greater cheerfulness of aspect has also been obtained in the new day-rooms than existed under the previous arrangements", an upgrade further "increased by the addition of decorations and objects of interest" (SCL 1878, xliv). The partition between the main gallery and the corridors was removed on the male side of the Ayr Asylum, which greatly increased the day-room accommodation for these patients (Tenth Annual Report of the Ayr District Asylum 1880, 39), and in the Haddington Asylum dark passages and partitions that "divided apartments unnecessarily" (SCL 1884, xxvi) were removed. This removal had the effect of permitting more light and air into the spaces, as well as creating more "elbow-room" for the patients. Similar alterations at the Stirling Asylum increased the space allocated to each person, as well as improvements in the sanitary arrangements (SCL 1884). At the Glasgow Asylum, the sitting-rooms in the asylum section were designed in an irregular shape, to induce the feeling that the patients were in a home "not of inordinate size" (Glasgow District Board Annual Report 1898, 6).

Interior decoration

Interior decoration is frequently applied to create affective atmospheres (Anderson 2009), with affect being the material connection between a number of different material and tangible and ideological entities or bodies (Sedgwick 1993). Thus, in order to induce an affective atmosphere into asylum space, whereby patients' emotional state and behaviour was affected (Anderson 2009), the Commissioners and district boards encouraged the introduction of particular furniture, fabrics, surface materials, colours, flowers, decorative objects and so forth in order to create a calming and more "home-like" ambiance (see Fig. 4.1).

A strong reliance on the affective effects of such objects and decoration are expressed throughout the archival documents. For example, the Midlothian and Peebles Asylum increased the "home-like aspect of wards ... by additions to furniture and the carpeting of several of the day-rooms and dormitories" (SCL 1878, xlii). Indeed, the Commissioners standpoint was articulated as follows:

> Considering the class of patients for whom the Institution exists, it might perhaps be thought that the furnishing and decoration had been carried to excess; but it is pointed out that the satisfactory condition of an asylum is greatly dependent on the influence which is exercised on its inmates by the circumstances in which they are placed. Experience shows that their behaviour improves with their surroundings; that, when these are comfortable and cheerful, there is less noise and excitement, less destruction of property, and less indulgence in degraded habits. (SCL 1878, xlii)

There was, therefore, a direct link identified between the introduction of various materialities for aesthetic enhancement and amusements, and the patient contentment and improved behaviour. The creation of such an atmosphere was believed to have a calming influence on the patients' often long-term surroundings. Time and again the Commissioners praised this aspect of the institutional spaces created by the district boards, commending, for example, "the civilising effects of floral decoration" (SCL 1876, xxvii) at the Ayr District Asylum, or the extension of the ornamental painting and papering of the walls and the additions to furniture at the Fife and Kinross Asylum. It was stated in 1877 that the decoration of the wards at the Roxburgh Asylum was progressing rapidly and was of a "highly satisfactory and tasteful manner" (SCL 1877, xxxvi). Similar improvements were made to the Perth Asylum, which included replacing worn-out furniture with new and comfortable items, in particular armchairs, which were reportedly "much liked by the patients" (SCL 1892, xxix) and said to increase their tranquillity and contentment:

> These, it is reported, have added greatly to the cheerfulness and comfort of the asylum, and have been appreciated by the patients. The asylum was found in excellent order, and the condition of the patients was in all respects satisfactory. (SCL 1891, xxvii)

Again, the Commissioners noted that the Stirling Asylum had done much "to add to the comfort and contentment of the patients" such as "repainting rooms, relaying flooring with pitch pine, procuring comfortable couches and a larger number of chairs, adding to the decoration of the wards, and by many other similar arrangements" (SCL 1891, xxvii). At the Ayr Asylum, the medical superintendent reported that "the internal appearance and comfort of the House is much improved by papering the walls with pretty lively patterns, hanging numerous coloured pictures, furnishing the windows with valances, and providing additional chairs" (Ayr District Board

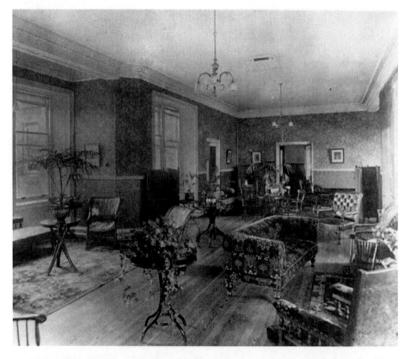

Fig. 4.1. Example of interior design: *Female Blue Room*, Inverness Asylum. The blue room was designed as a space where female patients could relax. The colour blue was chosen as it was considered to be calming. There was a similar *Blue Room* on the male side. Reprinted by permission of Scran Ltd.

Annual Report 1872, 15). In 1879 a "handsome carpet of good quality" was laid in the female day room, which was said to add "much to the comfort and appearance of the room" (Ayr Hospital Minute Book 1879, 8). In the early years of the twentieth century the use of pillows in the beds was commended, as well as the large number of easy chairs, which, "are said to be liked by the patients, and are believed to add to their comfort and peacefulness" (SCL 1903, xxviii). At the Haddington Asylum, it was reported that additions had been made to the furnishings, which included "chairs, rugs, tables, and small decorative articles" (SCL 1903, xxxiii), and improvements had been made to the dormitories such as reflooring in pitch-pine wood, as well as strips of carpet between the beds and blue blinds (as today, viewed as a calming colour) fitted to the windows.

As such, the villas were provided with sofas and easy chairs for comfort and contentment, a piano for entertainment, and pictures, plants and other objects for decoration, which all added to the cheerful and bright aspect of the wards. Within a year of opening, though, the *Evening Express* (1904, np) reported that the arrangements in regard to furnishings were not in "apple-pie order", and that the District Board should thoroughly investigate this claim, as the ratepayers were "entitled to know whether or not they have got good value for money".

Interactions between human bodies

Interactions between human bodies were also incorporated into the design of the asylum and were viewed as a powerful tool in the management of the patients. Through creating opportunities for human bodies to interact within the asylum through design and the formation of affective atmospheres, a *subtle* or "soft" control of patients within the asylum was made possible, rather than the mechanical restraint of previous years. The management of human bodies included the control and regulation of patients within the highly designed spaces. Furthermore, the creation of such spaces was expected to have the dual effect of not only resulting in an affective atmosphere capable of managing the asylum population, but also engaging the patients' minds by employing them in the construction of such spaces. As such, in the Roxburgh Asylum much of the construction work was undertaken by the male attendants and the patients together (SCL 1877, xxxvi) and the patients at the Banff Asylum were responsible for crafting the valances and rugs, which added to the "cheerful and comfortable appearance of the wards" (SCL 1883, xvi).

Again adding to the creation of a home-like atmosphere capable of affecting patients' behaviour, seating was arranged so as to have male and female patients alternating at the dining tables during meals instead of segregating the sexes (Haddington Asylum Patient Book 1868, np). It was noted as being implemented with ease into asylum arrangements, and was first trialled at the Haddington Asylum. Far from producing disorderly conduct, which was initially feared, the arrangement further introduced into asylum life a characteristic of ordinary life, and was praised as a useful tool in the management of patients. This set-up echoes Foucault's passage laid out in *Madness and Civilization* which explores how William Tuke, an 18th-century philanthropist and pioneer of moral treatment, forced maniacal patients to eat meals at the table with his family, "where everyone was obliged to imitate all the formal requirements of social existence" (Foucault 1965, 249). Similarly, the manner in which the tea was served at the Lanark Asylum was praised. At this institution, patients sat at "family" tables in the dining-hall, where tea was made in separate teapots for up to eighteen people: "the difference in the flavour of the tea thus infused is so remarkable, and its appreciation by the patients so evident, that a hope is expressed that all the inmates may in time be supplied with tea prepared in this way" (SCL 1905, xxxiv). Again, at the Glasgow Asylum, the crockery was admired as being "home-like ... free from any special institution design" (Glasgow District Board Annual Report 1898, 22). These dining-hall examples highlight the desire to bring into the asylum more "normal" objects and practices, creating a natural environment for the patients by implementing small gestures that closely match ordinary life, despite the wider institutional setting.

Regulation of encounters between human bodies also included patients meeting people they did not otherwise meet on a daily basis. Regular visits from authoritative figures such as members of the General Board and visiting medical superintendents were recommended as beneficial, "who should show himself to be in reality, as well as in name, the friend and guardian of the patients, and their shield and protection against the roughness and caprice of the attendants" (SCL 1873, lii). Additionally, ladies from Brabazon societies visited both the Midlothian and Peebles Asylum. These societies consisted of a number of local ladies from the nearby neighbourhood, who visited the asylum and engaged the patients in, among other activities, rug making, wood-carving, wood painting and bent-metal work (SCL 1900), and their visits were reported to "lend brightness and fresh interests to many of the inmates" (SCL 1911, xxxvi). These examples give a glimpse into the relationship between the institution and its neighbours, with a number of the locals taking an interest in the wellbeing of the patients through an early form of occupational therapy.

Afterthoughts

This chapter, taking inspiration from the geographical literature on affect, atmospheres and architecture, has recognised that a close, complete system of surveillance and management by the asylum staff was coupled with a sensibility alert to how the physical environment of the asylum buildings–with the capacity to cure, control *and* care–were viewed as a vital tool for the everyday running of the institution. Thus, the need to (re)create a tranquil, secluded and aesthetic yet still functional space through the creation of affective atmospheres, was recognised as a crucial component of the nineteenth-century asylum, affecting the physical and mental health of individual patients and also the management and treatment of the insane population as a whole. The creation and engineering of affective spaces was hence manipulated with the aim of managing the patients, although this was not often labelled explicitly as "management". The internal spaces were thus viewed as a powerful affective/effective tool over the patients, with the superintendents and Commissioners constantly engineering their layout, design and aesthetics to achieve improved behaviour, and hence a population that was easier to control. As such, it has clearly been shown that those in positions of power had the *potential* to consciously and politically manipulated behaviour (Sharp 2009), through the careful design of space.

The asylums constructed after the *Lunacy (Scotland) Act*, 1857, were one stage in a long trajectory of institutional design. The Scottish Commissioners in Lunacy and their contemporaries took inspiration from the buildings preceding the Act, learning from their deficiencies and manipulating designs to create buildings that would be fit for purpose. The buildings' goal was the safe incarceration of a specific population, but also they needed to be both functional and curative spaces, with the ability to exert diverse influences over the patients. Additionally, the buildings were designed to make the attendance, observation and nursing of the patients within the institution as efficient as possible, with the architecture and the staff working together to achieve two goals: the discharge of curable patients; and the creation of a homelike environment for long-stay, incurable patients. These goals, although arguably fitting together somewhat awkwardly, were designed to be realised through the engineering of the internal spaces to create a certain atmosphere.

Nineteenth-century authorities used and manipulated asylum spaces, therefore, to have the *potential* to affect institutional inhabitants, creating, they hoped, a curative machine through architectural arrangements. They organised the space, and the distribution of individuals within this space, to have therapeutic value, with the institution, rather than medical treatment (brought in later), being the remedial apparatus. The engineered spaces within the Scottish asylums studied should not, therefore, be configured as solely repressive devices, for they had the power to affect but also be affected (McCormack 2005) as they come in contact with other bodies and other affects.

Engineering affective atmosphere in asylums–Did it work?

The archival sources contained numerous reports about the positive effects of the design measures. Continual mention was made of improved behaviour; "less noise and excitement, less destruction of property, and less indulgence in degraded habits" (SCL 1878, xlii). Indeed, an exceptionally high recovery rate at Stirling Asylum was ascribed as a result of the environmental changes (SCL 1887). In 1903 the structural re-arrangements at the Midlothian and Peebles Asylum seemingly produced "a very marked improvement ... in the order and restfulness of the patients and in the smoothness of administration" (SCL 1903, xxxiv).

Emphasising the importance of subtle affective atmospheres as a tool for the management of patients, Sibbald (1897, 12) remarked:

> The removal of mechanical restrictions was the result of finding that most patients could be induced to submit to control when it was accompanied by efforts to gain their confidence by the exhibition of kindly sympathy and a desire to promote their comfort. It was found that the resistance of the patients to detention was, in most cases, diminished, if not removed, when it was made evident to them that those under whose charge they were placed were anxious to help and benefit them; and experience showed that the introduction of additional arrangements obviously intended for the advantage of patients, combined with the removal of irksome restrictions, had the effect of still further tranquillizing the patients and promoting their contentment.

These authors were, however, heavily invested in the asylum system. They needed to promote its success and champion their solution in the face of ever-increasing patient numbers. Sometimes, however, they let down their guard, demonstrating a rowing back from the asylum ideal *contra* to the surety of previous claims that the affective atmosphere of asylum spaces provided the best environment for the insane:

> We have become so accustomed to regard the gathering together of insane patients in large numbers in asylums, as the most appropriate manner of disposing of them, that we rarely pause to inquire the grounds on which this system has become so general. Nevertheless, it would not be easy to defend it, except on reasons of convenience and economy. Impassionately [*sic.*] and closely investigated, it bears in many respects the aspect of an evil; but an evil for which, under the circumstances of modern life, it may be difficult to find a complete remedy. (SCL 1870, xliv)

Despite this hint of uncertainty, the Commissioners, architects and media reports, most likely due to a lack of alternative solutions and huge investment in the asylum system, continued to promote the asylum into the twentieth century. The *Free Press* reported that the Aberdeen Board showed their awareness of the effectiveness and importance of engineering affective spaces when observing: "pleasant and comfortable surroundings have a marked influence in diminishing irritability and restlessness, and in contributing to the happiness of the patients" (*Free Press* 1904, np); and apparently the medical superintendent's motto regarding the asylum was "keep [it] lively and home-like" so that cure would result if it was within possibility (*Evening Gazette* 1906, np). The asylum superintendents and the Commissioners in Lunacy designed spaces to exploit the affective powers of the built environment through actively tailoring the asylum, creating an aesthetic capable of *potentially* affecting the behaviour and emotions of the patient, with the aim of either leaving the asylum cured and heading back into social and working life, or increasingly, remaining in the institution as good "workers" supporting the running of the institution. Ultimately, the asylum was designed to embody curative *and* caring potentials through architectural and interior design, either by restoring reason or at least by encouraging patients to act "sane" through recreating "ordinary" life.

To finish, therefore, following Kraftl and Adey's (2008, 219) caution that "there is not (and could never be) a neat or complete correspondence between the design of affect and its experience; the creation, evocation, and experience of affect is just not like that", as it is never certain how an individual will respond, this chapter recognises that spaces can only ever be engineered and designed to be *potentially* affective: there will always be "gaps" between the engineers' interior and how a building's dwellers experience, receive and respond to the affective atmospheres being engineered. Additionally, as there is, of course, "missing voices" in this study that have *not* been retained in the official records, but whose lives were, for better or worse, directly affected by the institutions that were constructed and the system that was created to manage this particular sector of society, the true affective power of the asylum will never be known.

Chapter Five

The Ghosts of the Refractory Ward: R.D. Laing and (Re)configuring Psychiatric Spaces of Care

Cheryl McGeachan

Introduction

One day I was called to the professor's office.

'I hear, Ronnie, that you see patients in front of your desk. Is that right?'

'Yes, sir.'

'I know you are very interested in patients but I just want to warn you–don't get too close to them'. (Laing 1985, 142)

The Scottish psychiatrist and psychotherapist Ronald David Laing (1927-1989), became internationally renowned for his work on humanist approaches to the so-called "psychotic" patient. In texts such as *The Divided Self* ([1960] 1969)*, Self and Others* ([1969] 1972) and *Sanity, Madness and the Family* ([1964] 1970) co-authored with Aaron Esterson, Laing frequently sought to convey the different spaces of "asylum" he experienced as a psychiatrist and that he later sought to create. By journeying through Laing's encounters with his patients in different spaces of Gartnavel Royal Hospital in Glasgow during the 1950s, this chapter seeks to reveal the differing ways in which Laing (re)configures psychiatric and therapeutic spaces. Through investigating *the rumpus room* experiment, this work will chart the importance of patients' experiences of architectural space had on Laing's re-envisioning of psychiatric practice and the spaces of mental health care. Attention will specifically turn to issues of environment and the complex interconnections between the spaces of care, the psychiatric encounter and the worlds of individuals experiencing mental ill(health).

The psychiatric encounter is intimately intertwined with the performative spaces of its creation and implementation (Morrison 2014). Bound up within a phenomenological and existential tradition, Laing challenged the traditional psychiatric encounter by offering alternative forms of practice and care that took various spatial forms. As the opening quotation demonstrates, Laing's desire to get closer to the patient (physically and therapeutically) was seen as dangerously transcending the boundaries of conventional psychiatric care. Recently, increased attention has been given to the life and work of Laing in human geography and beyond in order to tease out and illuminate the importance of his spatial approach to mental health care (McGeachan 2013, Miller 2004). However, despite this renewed attention little has been written to-date regarding his relationship to architecture. Recent scholarship within social and cultural geography has drawn attention to "practising architectures" (Jacobs and Merriman 2011) whereby *material matter* (walls, stairs, rooms, doors and corridors) sits intimately alongside *human mattering* signalling meaning and judgement (love and hate) but also affect and atmosphere. A key thread in these discussions is the idea of inhabitation and work has focussed upon the geographies of "being-in" architecture reminding us "that through the process of inhabitation building users, experts, material and immaterial things encounter one another in a myriad of complex, choreographers and unexpected ways" (Jacobs and Merriman 2011, 213; Lees 2001). Within the psychiatric encounter of the mental hospital, varying practices of spaces and experiences of inhabitation reveal themselves highlighting the "liquidity of architecture" (Cache 1995) and the different embodied, emotional and affectual experiences inhabitation can take.

Through exploring Laing's role as an "architect" of alternative psychiatric space, new insights into the making of such architectural spaces and the various ways in which buildings inhabit lives of patients and practitioners are revealed. This chapter begins by highlighting Laing's time spent in the female refractory ward at Gartnavel Royal Hospital in the early-1950s, demonstrating how the ward itself, and the people within it, influenced his theories and practices as a young psychiatrist attempting to find his place in the difficult arena of 1950's psychiatry. Following Laing's own experiences as a participant observer in the ward the affective powers of architectural atmospheres are highlighted in relation to sounds, feelings and bodily experiences. Following this, Laing's carefully devised architectural experiment, the "rumpus room", will be discussed in order to show how this work highlights his deepening awareness of environmental aspects and interpersonal relations in the world of the mental patients, also illustrating his awakening desire to (re)create psychiatric spaces of his own.

Navigating through Gartnavel's female refractory ward

When Laing returned from army service to Glasgow in November 1953 to complete his psychiatric training he was placed within the "Women's East" wing at *Gartnavel Royal Mental Hospital* (Andrews and Smith 1993, Morrison 2014). Gartnavel was a large, classic grand Victorian complex, built in the nineteenth century as an asylum (see Fig. 5.1). Wards were divided into the more wealthy fee-paying, "Gentlemen's West" and "Ladies West" with "Men's West" and "Women's East" for non-fee payers (Clay 1996, 53). This was a place that Laing had briefly visited during his medical training at Glasgow University, but the female refractory ward where Laing was to spend the majority of his time was a strange new environment that was considerably different from any other ward he had previously observed. This was Laing's first real experience of the world of the mental hospital, and the patients that he encountered here were not new psychiatric cases but chronic, long-stay patients, some "who had been 'in' for ten, thirty, sixty years: since the nineteenth century" (Laing 1985, 112), and this environment required much adaption on his part. The ward itself was an overcrowded and violent place, with windows frequently being smashed and patients often fighting with one another for the attention of the staff (Clay 1996, 54). The atmosphere was one of rising tension as the patient-to-staff ratio was becoming larger by the month and tempers of both patients and staff were beginning to fray. Andrews (1998, 122) notes that "patient numbers at Gartnavel were mounting throughout the 1950s, the Hospital's population topping the 900 mark for the first time in its history at the end of 1953 (the month after Laing's arrival) and reaching a peak of 979 patients in mid-1956". The incredible noise of the ward prompted an instant reaction from Laing, catching him off guard, as he became absorbed into the very distinct environment, atmosphere and culture of the refractory ward.

The peculiar nature of the ward led Laing to view the female patients in an unusual way as, for him, this was an experience that contained resonances of past psychiatric memories but that was in many ways notably different from before (McGeachan 2013). It was noted that:

> The ward was entered through locked doors, and housed about sixty women in cotton day dresses who were allowed no personal possessions–no underwear, no stockings, no cosmetics–and who were given weekly baths where they were scrubbed and dried before being out back in their cotton dresses (Clay 1996, 54).

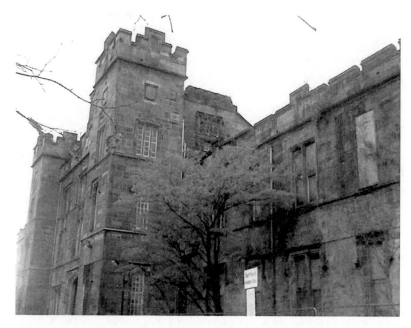

Fig. 5:1 Demonstrating the architecture of Gartnavel Royal Hospital. Photograph by Cheryl McGeachan.

On first sight these women appeared to Laing (1955) as "strange creatures" slipping in and out of view down the long narrow corridors of the ward, and they reminded him of Homer's description of the ghosts in Hades, "separated on their side from the living by the width of the Ocean, and, on the part of the living, by the Rivers of Fear" (Laing 1985, 112). For Laing, these women appeared to be distanced from him, not necessarily through their fragmented states, but because of a lack of understanding that he had about them. They appeared only to exist in a state of living-death, or to be "introjected" in clinical terminology, demonstrating their abstraction from the everyday world around them, and he struggled to find a way in which to describe these women:

> I wish someone could find a better name than introjected objects–ghosts, maybe; but they are not ghosts, either. (Laing 1967, 1)

Laing envisioned something in these women that did not lead them to be seen as frightening and disembodied, and he knew it would take time and effort, on his part, in order to discover what that something truly was. He set himself the question:

How can we entice these ghosts to life, across *their* oceanic abyss, across *our* rivers of fear? (Laing 1985, 112; emphasis in original)

In asking himself this question, Laing realised that the only way to uncover the nature of these female patients was for him to share their ward environment and attempt to become a spectator, but also a participant, in their semi-private worlds.

Gazing into the worlds of others–observing the day-room

In order to observe the patients in their own environment, Laing decided to spend two hours each day, for several months, sitting in the day-room and becoming absorbed into the daily lives of the women. Psychiatrist Harry Stack Sullivan (1955), an influential innovator in British psychiatry, noted that in order to find understanding the psychiatrist must become a participant observer in the world of the patient, and he was drawing heavily on the field of anthropology in his analysis. This method allowed the psychiatrist, in Sullivan's (1955, 381) mind, to engage with the patient more carefully, and he championed the notion of face-to-face or person-to-person contact between patient and analyst. Sullivan's conception of an interpersonal approach to psychiatry was highly influential on Laing's thinking about the importance of communication between patients and analysts, and his choice of method in the refractory day-room appears to echo Sullivan. The position in the day-room allowed Laing to become part of the "lunatic fringe of the psychiatric profession" (Laing 1984, postscript), spending as much time as possible in the company of patients one way or another and absorbing himself into the ward environment. This notion of being a participant observer in the lives of others meant that Laing could no longer only focus upon the patients' responses to the environment, or to one another, but he also had to develop an acute awareness of his own feelings and reactions in the space around him.

One of his first experiences in his period of observation in the day-room, one that made him particularly aware of his own position, was the starkly contrasting responses he felt towards his female, rather than male, patients. Previously Laing had only professionally come into contact with male patients, and he noted on his arrival at Gartnavel that he was "glad to be among women" after his spell in the army (Laing 1985, 112). Laing positioned himself in a chair in the middle of the day-room, which was a particularly unusual thing for a doctor to do at the time, possibly due to the massive workload that most doctors were facing. Laing noted:

> I think the first thing that happened to me when I had sat myself in a chair
> was that several patients fought each other to hug me or kiss me, to sit on
> my lap, to put their arms around me. They ruffled my hair, pulled my tie. I
> got my trouser buttons ripped open. (113)

Laing suddenly became aware of the physical reactions he had to face by
entering into the patients' space in the ward, particularly a women's space
as a male authority. The vigorous physical nature of the women's advances
provoked particular bodily reactions from him that he was unaware he
would have. In draft notes recalling his initial time spent in the day-room,
Laing commented:

> My first impressions therefore were mainly of my own reactionist anxiety at
> raw physical advances, aggressive and/or sexual on my body, and horror at
> the general dilapidation of many of the patients, their obscenity and so on.
> Sometimes I was so physically shaken that I had to leave after half an hour,
> to find myself trembling like a leaf. (Laing 1955, 3)

Laing felt extremely uncomfortable at the physical nature of the contact
with these women: when grabbing, climbing and clawing at him, Laing felt
compelled to recoil. Although he willingly entered into their environment,
when the patients pushed themselves into his private bodily space, he found
it so difficult to manage his own responses that, at times, he had to remove
himself completely from the day-room in order to regain his composure. It
took many of these encounters for Laing to become attuned to working with
these women in *their* environment, and it was the awareness of himself, and
his own bodily reactions, that he believed was essential in order to uncover
an understanding of the situation.

Laing's position in the day-room allowed him to immerse himself in the
atmosphere of the ward, and one aspect that particularly resonated with Laing
was the incredible noise that reverberated around the rooms. He noted:

> At first the ward sounded like an out-of-tune orchestra endlessly tuning up,
> each instrument unrelated and out of pitch. (Laing 1985, 114)

Each sound that was being produced appeared initially to make no sense
and seemed to clash with the other noises resounding in the room, but slowly
Laing began to notice a change in what he heard:

> With some acclimatisation, it began to dawn on me that the autism of each
> patient, although autistic, was interwoven with that of the others. A more
> appropriate analogy seemed with the illumination that comes when the jumble
> of sound in a difficult piece of music all suddenly makes sense. (114)

It became clear to Laing that there were patterns in the noise he was hearing and that, by spending the time actively listening and tuning himself into these sounds within the ward space, he could start to hear things that no longer simply represented noise, but that began to make some sense and fit together. The hours that Laing spent as a child learning to play the piano required him to train himself to listen carefully to the pitch of the keys, and here in the day-room Laing was implementing these skills once again in an attempt to uncover some of the hidden messages that he believed his patients were delivering to him through the sounds being made.

The noise and movement occurring in the day-room appeared in conjunction with the silent and insular nature of several of the patients. Many of these patients were overlooked at first glance due to their quiet status, and Laing (1985, 113) recalled how most of them "sat huddled in chairs, talking to no-one, not even themselves, being spoken to by no-one", appearing almost to be slowly sinking out of existence. These were the patients towards whom Laing would later be drawn, but it was clear that unravelling the stories of these women would be an enormously challenging task. It was only through time and perseverance in the day-room that Laing began really to see, to hear, to sense the environment here and, because of this, to start empathising with the people that existed in it. He noted:

> When the chaos within myself settled somewhat, I began to try and understand what was happening. I thought in psychoanalytic terms, and saw and heard examples every minute of regression, projection, condensation, identification, displacement, symbolisation etc. However, the way to relate oneself with psychotics is not through the head but through the navel, and when I actually began to perceive a little of their feelings, I began to find it increasingly difficult to comprehend with my head what was going on until I did not try to do so any more (Laing 1955, 3).

This gradual displacement of cognition/representation; attempting to tune in, bodily, to the immediate sights and rhythms of the room has resonances with the ideas surrounding *non-representational theory* (Lorimer 2007) and emphasises, one again, the intimate relations that exist between material matter and human mattering. Glimpsing the patients through the eyes of psychiatric theory left him unable to arrive at any form of convincing understanding of these people, and so he felt the need to form a relationship with them through utilising the space they were in which he could attach himself to their emotions. Laing appeared to be resisting the practice of seeing patients through a scientific gaze in favour of viewing them in human terms, and instead of distancing himself from the people he was treating he wished to push himself closer to them: a thoroughly spatialised practice of replacing distance with (sustained) proximity. By choosing to draw closer to the patients, Laing had to move away from the scientific approach and its particular way of viewing, and his position within the day-room gave him the opportunity to attempt this change in direction.

Mentoring Laing

Due to the complex nature of the situation he was seeing and the unfamiliarity of the female patient to him, Laing decided to change tack slightly and reach out for help to the only people he felt could contribute to the process of understanding the inhabitation, and so he called out to the patients themselves. Laing (1955) noted that at first it appeared that the patients were living in their own worlds, sharing them with nobody, but he began to notice that this was true only in a sense, as the environment of the ward was a collective one and there were people who could communicate their understandings of the situation with him (Laing 1985, 114). Laing became friendly with a small number of the women, who he called his "ward philosophers" (Laing 1955, 4), and in turn they gave him rare insights into the private worlds of their fellow patients. One of these women, to whom Laing became particularly close, was an older patient who had been hospitalised on a regular basis for over twenty years. This woman had spent the majority of her life, when not incarcerated, devoted to her mission work which was carried out with prostitutes in deprived neighbourhoods. She had been taken into psychiatric care with "episodic manic attitudes" in which she ranted, roared, and raved about the sexual horrors that she believed she had endured, sometimes at the hands of the ward doctors (Laing 1985, 112). Laing noted that she would constantly be moving, "pacing" or "prancing" around the ward floor (112). Once, when the woman approached Laing in his chair in the day-room, he asked her, "Why are you like this?" He recalled that she turned to him calmly and clearly replied, "Read Psalm 32, verses 3 and 4. I stuck at the Resurrection", and with this she continued her daily act of pacing and roaring around the ward (113). Later that day Laing looked up the verses that she had asked him to read:

> When I kept silence, my bones waxed old through
> my roaring all the day long.
> For day and night thy hand was heavy upon me:
> my moisture is turned into the drought of summer
>   (quoted in Laing 1985, 113).

The next time he saw the old woman he told her that he had looked up the verses up, repeating them to her, and he reports that she appeared touched by his gesture. In taking the time to listen to the woman, and also importantly to show that he had heard what she had said, Laing had opened up avenues of communication that had previously been closed and a relationship had been struck. Laing (113) recalled that at times she continued in her previous ways, but that:

> Most of the time she would sit down beside me and we would silently survey the scene together. From time to time, spontaneously, or when I asked her to, she would elucidate for me what this patient was doing, standing, immobile, all day, staring at the sky, and what that one was doing. She took me on. She became my mentor.

For Laing, this patient became his portal into understanding the seeming bizarre behaviour of the women in the ward. The woman would often explain to Laing the strange goings-on and allow him a rare glimpse into the daily workings of the patients' worlds. He recalled:

> She told me that that patient, for instance, huddled in the far corner of the ward, gazing fixedly out of the window, was furious that I had not looked at her when I entered the ward. That patient curled up under a table, she told me, had been playing at being a snake for years. (114)

What appeared at first to make no sense became much more understandable when seen through the eyes of the patients themselves. It could be viewed that Laing required this guide not only to help uncover the "mad" behaviour that he was seeing, but also to unravel the complexities of inhabitation in the refractory space. It could also be argued that, by singling out one patient and listening only to her responses without investigating this analysis further, Laing was only gaining a very restricted view of the refractory ward and its patients (Abrahamson 2007, 210). Although it is important to realise that his view of the ward was a limited one, Laing's desire to seek invitation into the worlds of his patients required him to gain knowledge of the female patients of whom he previously had little experience, and because of this he felt the need to rely on the patients themselves to help him to understand them and their unique use of their environment.

The "rumpus room" experiment

Driven to investigate further the development of relationships between patients and staff and the significance of particular hospital environments, Laing conceived an experiment that would explore what would happen if a small group of patients were placed together in a separate space and treated by the same nurses over a period of time. Although this particular project was essentially Laing's own architectural creation, similar group work with patients at Gartnavel had been carried out previously (Andrews 1998, 133). Through Laing's time spent observing the patients in the refractory ward, he had begun to question the role of the hospital environment and inhabitation experiences in the lives of the patients. For Laing (1957/1981, 20), the environment was a key therapeutic element in the treatment of patients and he argued that "we and the environment are in interplay from the beginning"; not only are we permeated by our environment but "our environment is outside, around, within us, it courses through us". It appeared to Laing that the environment of the refractory ward was not significantly therapeutic, and in order to foster meaningful relationships between patients and staff he believed that there had to be a change to the environment which they shared. The information about the physical design of the "rumpus room" is somewhat limited but it is documented that Laing took over the separate room in the ward for his experiment which was large, bright and newly decorated. The room was adjoined to a doctor's bedroom, kitchen and a staff billiards room, and a door leading from this set of rooms could be locked or kept open as required by the staff. Inside the room were materials for knitting and sewing, magazines and comfortable furnishings, all of which created a visual contrast from the minimal aesthetics of the host ward (Cameron, Laing, and McGhie 1955, 1384).

Laing chose eleven of the women in the refractory ward to be part of his experiment. The criteria for selecting these women centred upon their level of isolation from both the world outside of the hospital and the actions inside the ward itself. None of the eleven patients were able to leave the ward unless accompanied by their visitors, and the majority of the women selected were considered too "disturbed" to take part in any of the ward activities such as the hospital dances. All of the women chosen were diagnosed as schizophrenic, aged between 22 and 63 years, and had been residing in the same ward for over four years, without any remissions (Cameron, Laing, and McGhie 1955, 1384). The figure of the schizophrenic was becoming increasingly popular for research throughout the 1950s, acting as "a kind of test subject" for the many different psychotherapeutic schools all fighting to become the ruling body on the subject (Andrews 1998, 134). Alongside this was the belief that schizophrenia was an incurable illness, bringing with it a curiosity that compelled many new psychiatrists to take on this challenge in contrast to other stages in the history of psychiatry where this very incurability has arguably led to a shunning of the chronic, schizophrenic cases. Laing was one of these psychiatrists particularly fascinated by the complex nature of the schizophrenic patient, and his experiment aimed to demonstrate that an understanding of these individuals could be found through the relationships they make in particular spaces.

The results of the year-long "rumpus room" experiment[1] appeared in *The Lancet* in 1955 as part of a group of articles, entitled 'In the Mental Hospital', that were chiefly concerned with the value of work and active occupation in mental patients. The article, *Patient and Nurse Effects of Environmental Changes in the Care of Chronic Schizophrenics* authored by Laing, Cameron and McGhie, details the events that occurred throughout the "rumpus room" experiment and also shows the nature of the relationships between the patients and their nurses, including how they changed within the specifically designed room. Within the title of the paper the authors were keen to stress the centrality of the environment in their study. Laing and his colleagues (1955, 1384-1385) revealed that the events occurring on the first day became the standard procedure for the entire experiment:

> The nurses appeared for duty on the ward at 7.30 A.M. They shared general ward duties until 9 A.M. when they took their patients over to "the room" where they stayed with them until they took them back to the ward for lunch at noon, leaving them there, while they had their own lunch. At 2 P.M. they collected them again from the ward and took them back to "the room" until 5 P.M. The nurses then returned to "the room" for about half an hour to write up the day's happenings.[2]

The patients were spending five days a week, six hours a day, with the same set of all female nurses, and it was hoped that this would be an adequate amount of time for meaningful relationships to occur. It was recognised that at first the patients used the space inside the room as nothing more "than an extension of the ward" (1385), taking up positions within the room that were reminiscent of their use of space in the ward. The nurses attempted to utilise the material in the room and strove to encourage the patients to knit or draw, but they noted that even when they placed a magazine on a patient's knee they initially did not respond to it in any visible way. Throughout the day, though, the nurses noticed that a few of the women started to take part in small activities such as drawing or reading, but the majority still appeared indifferent to the activities on offer (1385). When the first day was over and the nurses took the patients back to the main ward, they described the way in which they all seemed to become absorbed once again in their long-standing customary roles, taking up the same positions in the ward that they had left that morning; and it appeared that nothing had really changed.

On the second day of the experiment, it was noted that the women were all waiting at the ward door, half an hour earlier than scheduled, to be taken across to the room, and Laing recalled how this was "one of the most moving experiences of my life" (Clay 1996, 55). For him, this was a symbol that there was something positive to be gained for the patients from this experiment, and he became convinced that there were more encouraging outcomes to appear.

The nurses were not so easily convinced, however, and they expressed great concern over their loss of control over the patients' movements. The nurses were consistently worried that the patients could run away while they were being taken from the ward to the special room, and they were afraid they could not "keep a grip on them" (Cameron, Laing, and McGhie 1955, 1385). There was a feeling of uncertainty from the nurses over how the patients would react to a new set of procedures, so their cautious approach to transporting the patients from the ward to the room highlighted their anxiety. Before moving the patients into the room, the nurses would heavily sedate them, and they always kept the stair door locked in case any of the patients attempted to escape (1385). If any of the patients did try to leave the room, the nurses would immediately run after them to bring them back due to their apprehension over what would happen if they got away.

As the research progressed, though the nurses slowly began to change their attitudes towards the experiment and its patients. The nurses agreed that there was indeed a gradual change occurring in how many of the patients behaved inside the room and their habitation patterns. Some of the patients began to use the material that was available, so they would read, sew or draw, and were doing so on a regular basis. Other patients would take over small jobs inside the room such as making tea or laying the table, and this became an important part of their daily activities. The nurses believed that their shifting reactions to the patients were ultimately due to this change in how the patients were behaving. The nurses became more relaxed in their approach, no longer feeling that the patients' movements needed to be so sternly regulated, albeit this was a steady progression. They began to sedate the patients less frequently and no longer consistently locked the stair door, allowing the patients to leave the room if they wished to do so. This free flowing movement outside of the room was allowed by the nurses' growing feelings of trust towards the patients. When the nurses had to leave the room to perform errands, the patients often followed them and sometimes they would help with the task that the nurse was called to do (Cameron, Laing, and McGhie 1955, 1385). The report noted:

> At first when patients left the room they had wandered erratically through the hospital, but now it was obvious that they were on their way to do something–to collect stores, to clean some part of the hospital, or to go for a walk in the grounds.

The patients were beginning to use the space of the hospital in different ways from before and were creating a wholly new micro-geography of "dwelling" in these spaces. Instead of moving aimlessly around the ward and wider hospital, they became more focussed due to the tasks in which they wanted to involve themselves, arguably rending more meaning to their everyday existence, creating an enriched "existential geography" (McGeachan 2014). Laing argued that these responses were indicative of the increased awareness that the nurses were gaining of the patients and their behaviour. The biggest change, Laing believed, lay not in the patients themselves, but in how the nurses were beginning to understand them. Laing noted that the nurses, in their weekly meetings with him, were beginning to report more phenomenological material and he recalled:

> They reported, for instance that Mary, who often stamped her feet and banged her chair on the floor was no so much angry, as they had hitherto supposed, but frightened–frightened in particular, of Peggy, who made friendly advances towards her, but which were taken by Mary as something more sinister. (Laing 1955, 7)

This attention to the particular detail of the patient was something that had been missing from the nurses' previous notes, and Laing (1955, 8) observed:

> There were now no tiresome stereotypes–"Mrs X has been uncertain today" etc. There was a spontaneous recital of the minutia and trivia of daily happenings, sometimes funny, sometimes boring, sometimes interesting, sometimes disappointing.

Laing argued that the nurse's relationships with the patients had developed to the point in which they no longer viewed them as simply another patient in the ward, but as individual people wrapped up in their own differing social and spatial situations.

Concluding remarks

The "rumpus room" experiment was developed on the premise of developing interpersonal relationships between patients and staff, ones that could be beneficial in developing understanding of the patient and their life-worlds. In order for these relationships to mature, Laing believed that a separate space needed to be created, away from the main ward, and therefore the room itself, for Laing, became a critical element in the experiment. That said, in the concluding discussion of the collaborative paper that was produced on the "rumpus room", the authors argued that "what matters most in the patient's environment is the people in it" (Cameron, Laing, and McGhie 1955, 1386) and the environment itself was placed by the wider team as a secondary element. Although the authors' placed the primary significance of the "rumpus room" experiment on the interpersonal connections that it fostered, Laing was increasingly insistent in later publications and interviews that the environment still had a key part to play in the developing of such relations (see Beveridge 2011). Unlike his co-authors, Cameron and McGhie in their follow-up work on this project, *Chronic Schizophrenia* (Freeman, Cameron, and McGhie 1958), Laing felt it was important to focus not solely on the patients themselves but on their "interpersonal microcosmos" (Laing 1990, 180) in order to gain understanding of their experience. This way of viewing the "rumpus room" connects directly to the non-representational enterprise of examining the lifeworld and the habituated nature of everyday existence (Anderson and Harrison 2010b). In emphasising the significance of understanding the patients experience from within and through their own worlds and networks, Laing is demonstrating a sensitivity to the unfolding nature of experience and the relationship between materiality and subjectivity (Wylie 2010) for everyone involved in the experiment. The women increasingly emerged as more rational and "sensible" in the nurses' non-representational account of "the minutia and trivia of daily happenings", willingly performing everyday tasks rather than their previous seemingly erratic behaviour (Cameron, Laing, and McGhie 1955, Laing 1955, 8).

The importance of the work of Maxwell Jones on *therapeutic communities*, although arguably underplayed by both Laing and Freeman at Gartnavel (Andrews 1998, 130-131), was highly influential to this experiment as it highlighted the "idea of the therapeutic community and of opening the doors" (Laing quoted in Andrews 1998, 130). With Jones' arguments in mind, Cameron and colleagues (1955, 1386) argued that the most significant element in the experiment related to the staff:

> It was the nurses. And the most important thing about the nurses and the other people in the environment, is how they feel towards their patients. Our experiment has shown, we think, that the barrier between patients and staff is not erected solely by the patients but is a mutual construction. The removal of this barrier is a mutual activity.

It was believed that during the experiment the patient's behaviour had altered and they had become more "social" than before, taking part in activities that required contact with others and spaces elsewhere in the asylum. Laing recognised the central importance of the Matron and nurses' roles and in a later interview claimed that "the nurses ran the whole thing" (Mullan 1997, 108), suggesting that his and the other doctors' role was secondary to theirs. Arguably, inside the 'rumpus room' there emerged a small community with certain individuals assigning themselves particular roles that allowed them to attach value to the material matter (room) and the human mattering (people, experiences, feelings) within it. This intimate relationship between "material" and "mattering"–architectural space and subjects–highlights the significance of the "room" to this experiment. As Severinsson and Nord (2015) have argued elsewhere, architectural space and artefacts–such as doors, walls, magazines, tables, knitting materials, etc.–become important incorporated elements into care model networks. For Laing (1985, 115):

> In that room, it became ever more clear to me that these patients were exquisitely sensitive to the nuances that some people never notice, or dismiss as petty. They are always there and far from petty. Most of us walk over them but some people drown in them, patients or not.

Undoubtedly, the "room" mattered in a variety of ways but especially in its ability to enable meaningful interpersonal relations to take place in multiple formations that Laing observed were not able to take place in the everyday refractory ward environment. Architectural design was therefore used as a device for encouraging positive relationships (Severinsson and Nord 2015, 140) but also for highlighting the nuances of mental ill-health that are often hidden in other hospital spaces.

As highlighted, throughout his psychiatric career Laing struggled to understand the experiences of mental ill-health and continuously turned to the environment and the architecture of the psychiatric encounter to reconfigure his understanding of his patients' worlds. This chapter has attempted to highlight the importance of material matter and human mattering to Laing's reimagining and reconfiguring of psychiatric space. Through examining Laing's time as a participant observer in the female refractory ward of Gartnavel Hospital and his designing of the spatial experiment the "rumpus room", insights into the ways in which meaning, affect and atmosphere comingle with core architectural features such as rooms, doors and walls come interestingly to the fore. Viewing Laing as an architect of alternative "asylum" spaces allows a routeway into thinking about inhabiting the mental hospital and spaces of mental ill-health that could usefully be further explored.

In returning to the "ghosts" of the refractory ward which led to the creation of the "rumpus room" experiment Laing (1985, 112) describes Ulysses meeting with his mother in the underworld:

> Ulysses goes to the land of the dead to meet his mother. Although he can see her, he is dismayed to find he cannot embrace her. She explains to him that she has no sinews, no bones, no body keeping the bones and flesh together. Once the life force has gone from her white bones, all is consumed by the fierce heat of a blazing fear, and the soul slips away like a dream and flutters in the air.

From this he interestingly (1985, 112) asks, "from what experience of life had that description come?", demonstrating his desire not only to understand the individual but to question their entire world from their experience of it. By engaging with the "ghosts" of the refractory ward Laing encountered, imagined and reconfigured real and meaningful spaces of care. During Laing's participant observation of the refractory ward he explored a range of multi-sensory encounters within the space, such as the acoustic nature of the ward and the raw, physical, embodied experience between himself and the patients, and sought to use this to formulate his own version of a caring place within the confines of the hospital. Jacobs and Merriman (2011, 214) consider an approach to inhabitation, drawing from Heideggerian principles, to be "dwelling or being *with*" buildings rather than a "dwelling or being *in*" buildings stressing that "[b]uildings inhabit our lives just as we inhabit them in an array of ways". By examining the "rumpus room" experiment and Laing's time spent observing the refractory ward from a "practising architecture" perspective this work has demonstrated the importance the patients he encountered during his work as a psychiatrist had on his (re)configuration of psychiatric practice and the spaces of mental health care. Issues of environment and the complex interconnections between the spaces of care, the psychiatric encounter and the worlds of individuals experiencing mental (ill)health have been central to the concerns of the chapter and illuminate possible ways forward for connecting geography and architectural concerns in new enlivening ways.

Notes

[1] The experimental room was named "the rumpus room" by the nurses, mirroring their ambivalence towards the experiment. However, after some time, when tensions became less, the name disappeared from use. (Cameron, Laing, and McGhie 1955, 1386).

[2] Despite thoroughly searching through the archival documents relating to the 'rumpus room' experiment, it appears that none of the notes compiled by the nurses remain.

CHAPTER SIX

NORMATIVE AND RELATIONAL ASPECTS OF ARCHITECTURAL SPACE: THE USABILITY OF COMMON SPACES IN ASSISTED LIVING FOR OLDER PEOPLE

MORGAN ANDERSSON

Introduction

Assisted living is an institutionalised type of collective housing for weak older individuals, with care and assistance provided within the facility (Schwarz and Brent 1999). Assisted living in Sweden forms a part of public eldercare, along with home-based measures such as home care. According to Swedish law, public eldercare is a municipal responsibility. The definition of assisted living may vary considerably between different countries, as does the organisation of eldercare, but there are some major structural similarities (Anderzhon, Fraley, and Green 2007, Regnier 2002, Zimmerman and Sloane 2007). An assisted living facility provides round-the-clock housing for the resident, often including care staff. As a rule, the facilities are subdivided into smaller residential groups with common spaces for social interaction.

The collective idea is thus present in the design of the facilities (Andersson 2013, Nord 2013b). In contrast to ordinary housing blocks, assisted living facilities belong structurally to an institutional, collective tradition, like prisons, hospitals and nursing homes (Markus 1993). A journey around Sweden visiting assisted living facilities reveals a variety of different architectural designs (Andersson 2011). However, to some extent this abundance is a chimera. A closer look reveals a striking conformity in the physical design in certain aspects such as the layout and types of rooms. Besides resident rooms there are normally corridors, a dining-room, a living-room and a common kitchen (Nord 2013b). Similar design models are also found in assisted living facilities in other parts of the world (cf. Regnier 2002, Anderzhon, Fraley, and Green 2007). Residents' apartments are often small, ranging from about 25 to, in exceptional cases, 45 square meters, containing an accessible bathroom, a small kitchenette and one, or occasionally two, living rooms. There are few rules concerning the physical design of assisted living in Sweden, however, those that do exist concern the provision of common spaces to make them legally a part of the residential environment. The rules were first introduced in 1993 (BFS 1993) and are still in effect (BBR 2015). They diverge from the building regulations for ordinary housing by allowing smaller apartments if the residents have access to common spaces:

> For a group of residents, rooms in the private apartments that relate to functions and equipment for cooking, daily social interaction and dining may be partly located to common spaces. The common spaces must have the size and functions to sufficiently compensate for the reduction in space in the private apartments. (BBR 2015, 54, my translation)

The use, or lack of use, of common spaces in assisted living or nursing homes has been highlighted as divergent from intended use, problematic and ambiguous (Hauge and Heggen 2008, Moore 1999, Nord 2011a, Andersson, Ryd, and Malmqvist 2014). Similar ways of apprehending use are a point of departure for this paper which aims to explore how usability of common spaces appears during the different phases in the design process of an assisted living facility: the planning, conception and use of the readymade buildings. A definition of usability in widespread use among researchers and evaluators is that the usability is "the extent to which a product can be used by specified users to achieve specified goals with effectiveness, efficiency and satisfaction in a specified context of use" (ISO 1998), in this case, architectural space in assisted living. Usability can be measured and evaluated (Warell 2001). However, when evaluations are carried out in real-life organisations and buildings, usability seem to defy efforts to find criteria and parameters for its evaluation (Blakstad, Hansen, and Knudsen 2008). Usability then appears as an effect of the user-environment interaction (Blakstad 2001), much more evasive and difficult to apprehend. The messiness in use, idiosyncrasy and the time/process component challenge the evaluators. It is argued that it is not possible to capture the ongoing changes in real-life use of buildings in an immobile image of usability, and the list of parameters is becoming longer and longer (Rasila, Rothe, and Kerosuo 2010). This discussion reflects these two different perspectives on usability. According to the first definition, usability is an idea of how a space is intended to be used, manifested in the planning and design processes. This represents normative aspects of space and of its *intended usability*. The architectural design of assisted living facilities often entails normative aspects of the built environment in the functional, aesthetic and technological senses. The normative aspects are here defined as the static, non-temporal or absolute representation of architectural design and spatial design as a "pattern" for any possible activity or action within it or in relation to it (Alexander, Ishikawa, and Silverstein 1977, 467). Once the physical layout of the building is set, it becomes a representation on a drawing. In the design of assisted living, normative usability may result in an architectural generality which counteracts personalisation of space and everyday practices, similar to the generality of other institutional environments (Goffman 1961).

In the second sense, usability is an ongoing process where negotiations between users and space produce new conceptualisations of space and thus reformulate the space itself. The normative aspects of the design are challenged by *relational space*, defined as the result of person-environment interactions over time, when the building is in use. The relational aspects of architecture are innumerable user-artefact constellations produced in the continuous use of the space (Yaneva 2009b). The relational aspects can be expressed as a production of "difference" or the emergence of "newness" (Anderson and Wylie 2009, 328).

Doreen Massey alerts us to the fact that "[c]onceiving of space as a static slice through time, as representation, as a closed system and so forth are all ways of taming it" (2005, 59). This corresponds to a normative interpretation of space, but, Massey suggests that the construction of space cannot be tamed. She argues that "what is, or should be, at issue in accounts of modernity and of globalisation (and indeed in the construction/ conceptualisation of space in general) is not a kind of denuded spatial form in itself (distance; the degree of openness; the numbers of interconnections; proximity, etc.), but the relational content of that spatial form" (Massey 2005, 93). This means that space is a result of all events and activities, or "[i]f we really think space relationally, then it is the sum of all our connections" (Massey 2005, 185).

As the continuous use of the environment produces complex new constellations between environment and users, differences appear between the normative planning context and the new context of use. The objective of this paper is to discuss this discrepancy between, on the one hand, the normative conceptualisations of space, in this case common spaces in assisted living, represented by the planning and design processes and, on the other, the relational processes of the continuous use of the spaces. This implies a discrepancy between an intended use of the spaces–a result of the planning and design processes–and their usability as an ongoing negotiation or performativity.

This paper is based on empirical data derived from a study of usability of common spaces in assisted living for older people. The study was conducted in 14 assisted living facilities in Sweden between 2009 and 2013. A mixed methods design was adopted. Individual, semi-structured interviews with residents and relatives were conducted, along with group interviews of staff. Observations were made in residential groups for older persons and in groups for older persons diagnosed with dementia. The observations were made at different times of the day over a one-year period. Finally, a self-completion questionnaire was sent to the staff (Andersson 2013, Andersson, Ryd, and Malmqvist 2014). The following narrative presents observations from this study.

A day at the assisted living facility

I am sitting in the common living room of an assisted living facility at seven o'clock in the morning. It is mid-December and pitch-dark outside. Two lamps in the large window are the only light sources. The staff return from the briefing in the staff room on the second floor. At twenty past seven everybody goes to the residents' apartments to assist some of them with their morning ablutions. Sounds are coming from the rooms–radios and televisions, someone screaming, conversations. Some doors are open, some are closed. Most residents are helped to the breakfast table in the common dining room. The very strong dome light is now on, producing a sharp, white light. The windows look like large, black mirrors. They arrive by means of wheelchairs and walkers, some with canes. At eight o'clock, a man from the technical department delivers the lunch canteens and the evening meals for the next two days. One of the staff members deals with it in the kitchen. At eight thirty, most of the residents are up and sitting around the dining tables. One of the staff is preparing the breakfast in the kitchen, whilst simultaneously keeping an eye on the residents in the adjoining dining room.

Breakfast is served at eight forty. Most of the residents are gathered. Some have their meals in their apartments and some are being assisted, either in the dining room or in their apartments. The staff talk to the residents, but the residents do not talk to each other. Subdued domestic sounds from the tables and from the kitchen accompany the meal. By nine thirty everybody has had their breakfast and the dining room is now empty. Daylight has arrived. Some residents have gone back to their apartments and a few of them are sitting in the drawing room. Some are away on communal activities. The TV is on. Between nine thirty and ten thirty the staff have their morning break and it is very quiet with nobody in the common spaces.

Coffee is served to some of the residents at eleven o'clock in the drawing room. They talk to the staff and to each other. By twelve o'clock, the washing up is done and the staff start helping residents to bathroom visits. After that, the majority have a rest in their apartments. At twelve thirty the staff start preparing lunch in the kitchen.

Lunch is served at one o'clock and all residents who can and want to, come to the dining room, either assisted or by themselves. The evening staff start at one o'clock and by two o'clock the dining room is empty. One resident returns from an outing with a relative: her son. The evening staff have their afternoon break at some time before four o'clock, when the day finishes. After that, they start helping the residents with their toilet routines and some of them are put to bed.

The evening meal is served at five o'clock. There are fewer residents in the dining room than at lunch. The residents continue to be helped to bed, while some remain in the living room watching TV. Some residents have visitors in their apartments. They stay for a short time. Coffee and sandwiches are served at about eight o'clock to those who want it and are still up. After the evening coffee it is very calm on the unit. Most residents have gone to bed. The last visitor leaves through the glazed entrance door. The staff finish between eight and nine o'clock, with the night staff arriving at nine o'clock. On this night there will be four of them in the building. After being briefed by the evening staff, the night staff return to the base unit. It is nine thirty in the evening and all residents are in their own apartments, sleeping or watching TV.

The lighting is in subdued night mode. Faint sounds from TV-sets. The first night round is made between nine and ten o'clock. It is quiet. At three o'clock the staff do a more extensive round. Nappies are changed and the residents are given some water or lemonade. The last round at five o'clock is a check-up. Only occasionally are there alarms from residents during the night. The staff watch TV or read. The most tiring period is between four and six o'clock. Then it starts all over again with a new day beginning at the assisted living facility following a similar pattern of use.

Use of common spaces in assisted living

The above narrative shows both major variations in the use of the common spaces throughout the day and a differentiated degree of use of different rooms in the unit. The common spaces were mainly used during mealtimes and in-between they were largely empty. Interviews revealed a discrepancy between the imagined and expected use of the common spaces and the actual use. There seemed to be certain expectations that the common spaces should provide the space for a satisfactory everyday social life. Quotes below express a desire to take part in a social community and, perhaps, disappointment when confronted with the blank reality that many of the residents were unwilling to socialise:

> It is important that we [the residents] can come together and have common meals and other activities in the common spaces. It strengthens the community. But when they have had their meal, they all go back to their rooms. You seldom see anyone out here. (Male resident, aged 89)

> Mum tried to spend time in the common spaces but she thought it was pointless because all the others were so tired and sick. The staff were more company for her. I think she had hoped for more social life in the assisted living facility. (Son, aged 69 with mother recently deceased in an assisted living facility)

The staff also expressed expectations that the common spaces were provided for the sake of the residents' social life in the unit and that the carers' task was to encourage them to use that opportunity, though often in vain as this did not seem to be attractive to all residents:

> To get them [the residents] to the common rooms, you have to persuade them. There is always a telephone call to make. They want to be in their own room. They sometimes visit each other, but not often. It is all about attitudes. We try [to make them come to the common spaces] but it depends on who is there. (Female carer)

Use of the different common rooms varied. The dining rooms were the most used, since the common meals are a recurrent and seemingly significant part of the residents' everyday lives; most residents have their meals together. The sitting rooms were used to a very low degree by the residents. Some of the people used them to watch TV at night. The study showed that the sitting rooms were used significantly more by the residents living in groups for older persons diagnosed with dementia. The difference in use between somatic and dementia units was acknowledged in staff interviews, revealing that the staff members identified a difference in the residents' experience and perhaps their perception of home:

> They [residents with dementia] are always with us in the sitting room. It is almost as if it's even more their home in the dementia unit. In the somatic [unit] they go to their rooms. They don't feel comfortable out there [in the common rooms]. They go to their rooms, so there is a difference. (Female carer)

In the non-dementia residential groups there were no residents in the sitting rooms and the dining rooms between meals; i.e. most of the time. In residential groups for persons diagnosed with dementia, residents occupied common spaces all the time; watching TV or just sitting there. Many residents with dementia also wandered around; a phenomenon that is well documented in persons with dementia (Algase et al. 2010).

The distinction between residents' home space and the staff's workplace appeared most clearly in the use of the common kitchens. The common kitchens were only used by very few residents on rare occasions, with the overwhelming majority of residents never using them. The majority of the residents, as well as the staff, considered the kitchens to be the staff's workplace rather than a part of the residents' home environment, although according to the regulations (BBR 2015), the kitchens are formally a part of the common spaces:

> Their apartment is their home. Kitchen and dining room is our workplace. There is a border between the apartments and the other spaces. (Female carer).

The residents' apartments were clearly demarcated as the private and secluded home space in interviews with both residents and staff. A female carer said in interview:

> Yes, their apartment is indeed their home. The sitting and dining rooms are theirs too but it's not private, it's common. That way it's not their home because they share it with others. (Female carer)

The apartment was the space that was by far the most used by the residents in comparison with the other spaces. It was also considered to be the most private space by both residents and staff.

The different uses of the rooms in the assisted living unit reflect private and public aspects of all spaces in assisted living for older people. They can be depicted as dichotomous opposites and must be understood in both a normative and a relational sense. Between these dichotomous extremes we can imagine a continuum of private or semi-private functions (see Fig. 6.1). The normative sense is represented by what physical properties and functions a space contains; what its ascribed private or public purpose is. The relational sense is decided by those who use it, which likewise determines the position of a specific space in the continuum. Both perspectives go against the legal prescription that all space is home space and, hence, private, according to the buildings regulations (BBR 2015). Common rooms are ambiguous in the sense that they are part of both the private and public spheres, thus affecting the use of the space as a home environment. Kitchens are most clearly the space identified by both residents and staff as a workplace and not home space at all. The dining-room was more easily defined as an extension of the apartment or the private sphere while the living-room was more ambiguous in this respect and could not compete with the privacy of the resident's apartments. While the staff were of the opinion that common rooms should be used by the collective, most of the residents preferred to spend time in the room they clearly identified as their private space, their apartment. The embedded ambiguities position the common rooms in an indistinct location in the private-public continuum (Andersson 2013, Hauge and Heggen 2008), or in mixed fractal configurations in which private appears in the public and vice versa (Nord 2011a). This potential gives rise to conflicts and awkward situations (Moore 1999).

What many institutional environments, including assisted living, have in common is that many of the actions normally performed in the privacy and seclusion of the home are carried out in common spaces (Goffman 1961). The individual has to adapt to this situation in which the physical closeness to fellow residents, who are strangers, may be equal to the physical closeness they would normally reserve for their intimates. People who have no connection with each other, apart from living in the same assisted living facilities for older people, have their meals together in the common spaces. Some people may feel comfortable with the situation and others not. The perceived sense of privacy is related to access, control and agency (Nord 2011a). Who can get into your room? Do you have control? Can you decide who can enter? Sommer (1969) describes how people create "micro-spatialities" of privacy in public or communal rooms. The boundaries of the private sphere are relational. A person with normal cognitive abilities can cope with different situations. For a person with limited cognitive abilities, caused by dementia for instance, this oscillation between different situations may pose a problem. This is often the case in assisted living.

Lefebvre's spatial concepts

In order to understand the mismatches, incongruities or creative use of space sketched in the narrative above in relation to design work, this paper will use the triad of spatial concepts defined by the French sociologist Henri Lefebvre (1991). The concepts represent three dimensions of space and all of them incorporate social and temporal aspects.

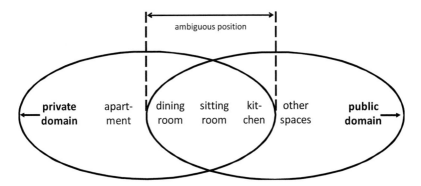

Fig. 6.1. The ambiguous position of the common spaces embracing both private and public domains. Diagram by Morgan Andersson.

The first concept is *spatial practice*. This dimension is the *perceived* space or the realised space. It is tangible, material space in the form of the built environment that constitutes the prerequisites for use. Perceived space implies a reproduction of social relations and societal values, spatial orders and institutional practices:

> Considered overall, social practice presupposes the use of the body: the use of the hands, members and sensory organs, and the gestures of work as of activity unrelated to work. This is the realm of the perceived (the practical basis of the perception of the outside world, to put it in psychology's terms). (Lefebvre 1991, 33)

The second dimension is *representations of space*. This is the *conceived* space or the image of space. This is the conceptualisation, knowledge and discourses of space of a cadre "of scientists, planners, urbanists, technocratic subdividers and social engineers" (38). This is linked to the means of communication such as the architect's drawing in the design process in which the imagined use of space is embedded. Lefebvre describes conceived space in terms of a void that facilitates socialisation:

> Empty space in the sense of a mental and social void which facilitates the socialization of a not-yet-social realm is actually merely a representation of space. Space is conceived of as being transformed into 'lived experience' by a social 'subject', and is governed by determinants which may be practical (work, play) or bio-social (young people, children, women, active people) in character. (33).

The third concept is *representational spaces*. This dimension is the *lived* space where space provides an existential context in which meanings and values are created by the individual(s). It is also where a space becomes a place; or, place as an effect of space and meaning. Lived space represents the dimension of *use*. Or described by Lefebvre, it is "space as directly lived through its associated images and symbols, and hence the space of 'inhabitants' and 'users'" (39).

What happens if we apply Lefebvre's triad of spatial concepts to a discussion about usability and the design process of assisted living? Is it possible to understand the equivocal use of spaces with the analytic support of these dimensions of space? In all three spatial concepts we can discern social and temporal mechanisms constituting the prerequisites for perceiving, conceiving and living space. The same mechanisms are relevant to the sequential stages of the design process; planning, construction and use. This discussion will reveal that Lefebvre's conceptual triad represents different dimensions of the same space.

> [S]patial practice, representations of space and representational space contribute in different ways to the production of space according to their qualities and attributes, according to the society or mode of production in question, and according to the historical period. Relations between the three moments of the perceived, the conceived and the lived are never either simple or stable" (46).

They coevolve in a dynamic and dialectical relationship as is suggested by Harvey (2006).

Architectural space and usability in the design process

Lefebvre's second concept, *representations of space*, invites an understanding of the design process through its focus on representations which are a prerequisite in the design dialogue and the realisation of ideas. The first stage of the design process is planning, in which the image of space is elaborated and developed as it is *conceived* by the actors, in this case architects and other professionals representing the commissioner, the municipality. The design process results in the blueprint of the building; the drawing or the model in which the intended use of the spaces is contained. It represents the normative "picture perfect" of the ideal building where the usability of the spaces is optimal. It is the *representations of usability*.

However, the design process is a messy and complex process, starting with thoughts, ideas, sketches and drawings. Planning is an incremental process involving clients, architects, planners and contractors (Ryd and

Fristedt 2007). The idea of the building is not *one* idea; it is the ideas of many different actors and users. It is a social process which derives from different sources of knowledge, the result of inputs from many persons and thus the product of innumerable interactions and negotiations during the design (Yaneva 2012). The architect's innovative and artistic work merges with the prospective users' imagined needs, the requirements of the client and the legislative apparatus. Different ideas are discussed and different solutions are proposed and rejected. The ideas of many different buildings also feed into the design process, for instance when the design team visits other buildings for inspiration and knowledge gained during the design process. According to Lefebvre (1991, 33), "spatial practice ensures continuity and some degree of cohesion". A repeated design model transfers ideas and practices from preceding buildings to the new ones: "this cohesion implies a guaranteed level of *competence* and a specific level of *performance*" (33, italics in original). The design of assisted living in Sweden and elsewhere is strongly associated with an institutional tradition of caring for the old, poor, weak and sick (Åman 1976, Markus 1993). There seem to be reasons to assume that this tradition is very vivid and still governs the design of most assisted living facilities today. This can be interpreted as a *spatial practice,* the first of Lefebvre's concepts. In a design perspective this is the existing realised, materialised space, the *perceived space*, informing new designs.

The normative aspects of architecture emerge when the architect visualises the result of this process in the form of an interpretation of the process and of the different actors' ideas of space in sketches and models. At this point it is possible to imagine the complete building and what it will be like to use it. This normative usability is eventually nailed to the product when the drawings and other construction documentation are produced. The drawing as a representation can be said to be a means to tame space, "a static slice through time" and "a closed system" (Massey 2005, 59). The drawings conceal the fact that the process of planning and constructing a building is a creative process to which a number of actors have contributed.

A significant *spatial practice* in the design process is the realisation, in which the building becomes a manifest, perceivable structure, still "tamed" in the words of Massey (2005). The representation of space–the drawing–becomes a building, in this case the assisted living facility. The construction materialises the many merged ideas into a physical and tangible space. The creative side of the architecture is that common spaces are often given varied and individual forms, whereas the architecture of the private residential rooms is similar in size and form, indicating that common spaces are ascribed greater importance in the daily life and care in the assisted living facility than residents' private rooms (Nord 2013b). Otherwise, the constructed space primarily follows the repeated structural scheme of division into units (or groups), horizontal communication areas (i.e. corridors), common spaces for collective activities (i.e. kitchen, dining room and sitting room) and rows of small residential rooms. One architect interviewed in the study articulated the intentions of this design model:

> The physical environment in assisted living has two purposes: A good home for the individual and room for social interaction. I think these purposes are equally important. (Female architect and researcher)

At this stage, the normative usability is transformed into real matter. Using the Lefebvrian concepts, the physical structure is *perceived space*, containing the prerequisites for use within a manifest form, presenting the *perceived usability* of the space as materialised, embedded normative ideas of the space. In the material space it is the architecture or the physical environment that sets the parameters for the intended usability of the spaces. The physical layout of the building limits what it is possible to do. The time between the production of the blueprint and the completed structure means that prerequisites often change and people involved in the design process change or are replaced. A number of researchers have long been advocating better briefing processes in order to accommodate alterations as a means of achieving better design and more satisfied users (Barrett and Stanley 1999, Blyth and Worthington 2001, Ryd and Fristedt 2007, Walker 2015). The physical layout of the spaces may no longer be congruent to the blueprint. Necessary adaptations are continuously being made in the construction process. Moreover, the blueprint does not contain the materiality of the completed building. The process thus produces different, or new, materialities as a result of temporal and social mechanisms (Anderson and Wylie 2009). Architecture is not created once and for all, "but is instead continuously transformed by the uses to which works of architecture are put" (Granath 1991, 55). The entire design process implies minor or major alterations over time. The last step is when the building is taken into use. When this happens perceived space links the representations of space (the blueprint) with the experience of space, lived space. Lived space sets aside the fact that the building itself contains the physical limitations for any possible use. The materiality of space becomes subject to negotiations of newness (Anderson and Wylie 2009). In the course of time, there may be new users and new needs.

Lefebvre's third concept, the *representational spaces,* is also called *lived space*. Well, how do we *live* space? When individuals live space, personal skills, characteristics and competences emerge from interaction with space and with other individuals (Wylie 2010). Thrift (2008, 98) recognises this space as mobile, "arising out of multiple encounters", an open-ended space of unlimited possibilities. Living in and using space continuously produces new and different situational configurations between space and users, in unexpected and sometimes chaotic processes (Anderson and Wylie 2009).

Normative usability is present in the explicit expectations for the social environment in assisted living of residents and others, as described earlier in the narrative above. An underlying appreciation seems to exist that collective activities are positive and that there is a need for some sort of social connectedness, represented by an idea of a community (Moore 1999) or the acknowledgement of the importance of common meals (Frankowski et al. 2011, Mol 2010). This is visible in architectural form. However, this idea of collective is, to a great extent, challenged by a life in space which counteracts a functioning community as defined by the blueprint. The residents are often too sick to socialise with others and their desire to socialise might be affected by the fact that they have no connection to their fellow residents, apart from having their apartments within the same group of residents. The use of the common rooms is substantially less than is expected and for which they were designed. Newness appears as empty common spaces in which the material bodies of residents are absent and, as articulated in some of the quotes in the narrative, desired fellowship (cf. Anderson and Wylie 2009). The usability of these rooms can also be seen as a product of the users' disparate understanding of their use in an ambiguous social context (Moore 1999). Taking into account these observations, it is not farfetched that an architect who was interviewed had doubts about common spaces:

> I have always thought they [common spaces] are difficult to design. They are so little used. It is difficult to socialise. Most of them [the residents] are in their rooms. They [the staff] wheel the sick out there to watch TV but they are often too sick to comprehend what is going on. (Male architect)

Or the residents who are healthier leave out the commonality offered in the public space since they identify weaker residents as being difficult to communicate with (Nord 2013a). The fact that residents choose to spend more time in their private rooms, avoiding the common rooms, seems to indicate that their wishes and needs may not have been taken into account in the design, with the consequence that use developed differently to that suggested by the normative usability. A reason for this could be that assisted living traditionally incorporates a "medical model" for care which influences the architectural design (Nord 2013b). This is valid for many national contexts (Schwarz 1997), and contributes to preserving assisted living as an institutional form of care as the attention of architects and planners is drawn to medical aspects. Less attention is consequently paid to the residential perspective and social aspects. This could explain why apartments in assisted living facilities are much smaller, compared to ordinary housing facilities. This is, however, contradictory since the residents are very old, frail and often suffer from a variety of disabling and painful conditions. The medical model has then failed to recognise that their private rooms are a place for many hours of necessary rest and that the commonality of assisted living is out of reach for these old residents. The complexity of this issue links to the Lefebvrian body–the spatial body–that is never inscribed in a uniform practice or incarcerated in a closed system of use (Simonsen 2005). The old bodies in this case produce their space by strategically resisting and benefiting from the affordances provided by space. The usability of the small private rooms should perhaps have already been defined differently at the blueprint stage, taking into account the choice of residents to stay in their apartments rather than in the common rooms.

The above narrative also indicates that the usability of the common spaces is related to negotiations of private and public aspects of everyday life. The degree to which these spaces are part of the residents' "home" is indeed a prerequisite for their use and perceived usability (Andersson, Ryd, and Malmqvist 2014). It seems as if the residents used their private rooms according to a scheme of private/public in which the common rooms were ascribed public qualities that did not coincide with the normative usability of an open and accessible collective. The avoidance of common spaces suggests that the residents refrained from using the whole assisted living facility as a home, which it *de facto* is according to the law.

Concluding notes

Usability appears in various degrees and guises in the design process of assisted living, including the last phase, i.e. the buildings in use. It emerges in normative and relational senses throughout the whole process. The usability of space, whether it is conceived, perceived or lived, is a social process. These processes do not occur "in the space", but "define" the space (Harvey 2006, 121). This also means that usability is defined by space.

The normative usability occurs when planning produces conceived space, composed of ideas of what an assisted living facility is and should be. These ideas govern the design as they become manifest in the representations–the drawings-produced in the planning process. The expectations of usability held by the actors, in this context primarily the architects, other construction professionals and assisted living staff, are transformed into something conceived and something perceivable: the physical construction producing a building. A basis for this is the architects' knowledge about what space is, about physical dimensions and laws, producing a general idea of usability; the *representation of usability*. This is also a social process of compounding individual knowledge or general knowledge within a group or society producing a normative space. A relational process is transformed into normativity including the personal experiences of architects.

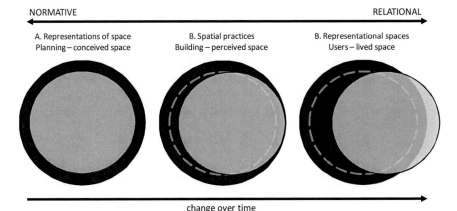

NORMATIVE   RELATIONAL

A. Representations of space   B. Spatial practices   B. Representational spaces
Planning – conceived space   Building – perceived space   Users – lived space

change over time

Fig. 6.2. A represents the normative planning context where the intended use (grey) is contained within the physical layout of the building (black). B shows how differences between the planning and construction phases produce new relations between the physical layout and the actual use. C shows how the interaction between the users and the environment produces new constellations between the physical layout and the actual use. Modified version of diagram from Andersson 2013.

The normative usability is challenged in the final phase of the design process; the use. This is lived space which is the space that *is* not, but *becomes* in the interaction between persons and space. This is space in becoming materialised by social and temporal mechanisms where *usability is created,* in ongoing practices, in unexpected enrollings, in interactions, in use. When facing this kind of usability, evaluators may run into problems since lived space is very difficult to "tame", to capture in a list of parameters and categories (Rasila, Rothe, and Kerosuo 2010, Massey 2005). However, the palette of usability and use is extremely varied and unpredictable. Since lived space is related to the experiences, preferences and actions of all sorts of emergent users, normative usability also occurs as expectations in continuous use. The normative usability embedded in space in the early design phases constitutes a promise that lived space in use might have difficulties in fulfilling.

There is an underlying conflict between how architecture is conceived and perceived on the one hand and how it is lived on the other. This conflict is time-related, since the process is repeated over and over again. Assisted living facilities are constructed over and over again in similar editions. Usability occurs as a mobile phenomenon moving further and further away from its incarceration in perceived space (Fig. 6.2). This iteration both conserves and provides the possibility for newness to occur. Not in shocking, revolutionary happenstances, but in small, incremental steps over time, questioned and challenged by the actors and users: "sometimes that-which-repeats-itself also transforms itself. Because each iteration occurs in an absolutely unique context" (Bennett 2001, 40). This suggests also person-related and non-temporal relations, since different individuals form exclusive connections to the same space at any moment. Assisted living as space is a result of all events and activities, whether it is conceived, perceived or lived.

CHAPTER SEVEN

TRANSLATING SPATIAL EXPERIENCES OF A MENTAL HEALTH CENTRE TO DESIGN RECOMMENDATIONS: A MISSION IMPOSSIBLE?

EBBA HÖGSTRÖM

> A building is made up of other spaces within it that move and change, even if its own walls remain fixed. (Grosz 2001, 7)

This chapter relocates to the mid-1970s in Sweden, to Saltsjöbaden in the municipality of Nacka, east of Stockholm, and to a newly opened outpatient clinic for mental healthcare. The clinic, *Saltsjöbaden Mental Health Centre* (SMHC), was one clinic out of three created in the pilot scheme *The Nacka Project 1974-1979*, an influential "actor" in the decentralisation and de-institutionalisation of Swedish mental healthcare.[1] The project was expected to provide "improved possibilities to reach goals such as closeness, accessibility, early interventions, continuity, flexibility and co-operation with other care providers" (Berggren and Cullberg 1978, 17). The spatial organisation and design of SMHC was anchored in these expectations, encompassing the dual aims of preventing people from becoming long-term psychiatric patients and fostering a culture of co-operation among staff. With its huge multi-functional waiting room, staffroom-cum-office without individual desks, non-personalised counselling rooms and lack of corridors, the mental health centre's spatial organisation and design was unique among outpatient clinics at the time. However, experiences of the architecture differed; it was embraced by many for its innovative and supportive design, whereas the design was criticised by others. Some years later, when SMHC was used as a precedent in guidelines for "the new psychiatry" by *The Swedish Health and Social Care Institute for Planning and Rationalisation* (SPRI 1985), most of its place-specific aspects relating to care ideology, work organisation and staff experiences were not brought to the fore. Why was this so? Why, in many ways, did these newer recommendations propose quite a different mental health centre to that programmed by the management of SMHC and experienced by staff and patients?

In this chapter, I use the case of SMHC as an example for examining difficulties arising in: (a) conveying architectural intentions when a particular spatial organisation is taken into use and merged with everyday practices and experiences; and (b) translating specific spatial experiences into general recommendations. I discuss whether it is possible to represent spatial experiences with the aim of influencing future spaces if their representation means that such experiences are easily "lost in translation". The theoretical approach derives from a relational-material ontology in which dimensions of process, experiences and differences form a core part in how space is conceptualised (Thrift 2006, Crouch 2010). In particular, the concepts of *event*, *spacing* and *representation* (Anderson and Harrison 2010a, Beyes and Steyaert 2011, Doel 2000) are used as tools in the present analysis.

SMHC operated during the era of Swedish mental healthcare decentralisation, when mental healthcare issues were part of public debate, psychiatric institutions were heavily criticised (Ohlsson 2008) and the will to test other ways of organising care and doing therapy was strong. Most of the reports from this period focus on organisational scale or therapeutic issues, which makes the case of SMHC important as a "close-up" of spatial and material everyday practices characteristic of an emergent decentralised care. This chapter thus focuses on micro-scale negotiations between preconditions ("raw" space), intentions (programme), configurations (design), experiences (use) and devised space (guidelines), addressing their intertwined influences in performing care. The empirical material presented in the chapter originates from a larger inquiry into the decentralisation of Swedish mental healthcare 1958-1995 (Högström 2012). The study comprised interviews, mainly with staff with direct experience of mental healthcare facilities in Nacka and, in particular, the Nacka project 1974-1979, but also with service users, relatives, architects and facility managers. Other methods used comprised documentary studies and the analysis of visual images and architectural drawings.

Spacing events–(re)presenting space

All events take place somewhere. The mutual influence of activity and physical environment, the *taking place*, and the concept of *event* are both central to a non-representational theoretical approach, especially in relation to orderings and change, and they open up ways of thinking about activities, experiences and objects (procedures, routines, rhythms, lightings, smells, sounds, material tactility, buildings, rooms, furniture etc.). An event can be material deterioration–for example, frequent use of a sofa wearing out its upholstery–or affects, maybe bodily movements such as sitting on the same sofa or something a person suddenly does (e.g. talking, walking), that alter future possibilities of doings and thinkings. Anderson and Harrison (2010a, 20) stress the event "as a continual differing, if only in a modest way, that takes place in relation to an ever-changing complex of other events". Materialities in this relational-materialist analysis of the social are not just "brute matter" (walls, doors, floors, glass, concrete, wood etc.) external to the more unconcrete event. Even if they differ in duration and solidity, they are as real or unreal as "apparently "immaterial' phenomena like emotion, mood and affect" (Latham and McCormack 2004, 705). Materiality is thus co-constitutive with immateriality, "an argument for apprehending different relations and durations of movement, speed and slowness rather than simply a greater consideration of objects" (705).

The taking-place, the event, is entangled with space or, better, with spac*ing*. In this connotation dimensions of process, experiences, differences and multiplicity are at stake, rather than just seeing space as a fixed and discrete frame of reference (Deleuze and Guattari 2004, Jones, McLean, and Quattrone 2004, Thrift 2006, Crouch 2010, Beyes and Steyaert 2011). Using the word *spacing* is thus part of an epistemological displacement, a changing viewpoint from objects to "doings", to a "processual performativity of space" (Beyes and Steyaert 2011, 52). Doel (2000, 125) argues that there is no space "behind" something (absolute space), nor space "between" (relative, relational, dialectical), but instead just spac*ing* (differentials). Every ordering is thus a momentary articulation rather than a fixed and external point, "not pointillistic but articular" (126).

If events are viewed as transient, fluid turning points, always taking place somewhere and complicit in spacings, and if the latter are non-tangible and differential, how could such processes/experiences be enabled, sustained and also passed forward? Passing experiences forward is an act of "assembling and dissembling" incessant habitual events and spacings with the help of any devices or means capable of translation (Dewsbury et al. 2002, 438). From a non-representational viewpoint, representations are transformers, and as such performative actions themselves. Representations are never "true" to the precedent that they are intended to represent and should be regarded as *presentations* enacting worlds as things and events, "rather than being simple go-betweens tasked with re-presenting some pre-existing order or force" (Anderson and Harrison 2010a, 14). Seen as performances, as doings, attention is altered from asserted meanings towards the material forms and conduct of representations (Dewsbury et al. 2002).

To *(re)present* is thus a transforming activity, working back and forth, as something that is given back, perhaps in another form, to what was once given to the senses (cf. Doel 2010). However, adopting such an experience-based and reciprocal approach to architecture defies the conventional knowledge base for architectural education and practice (cf. Cuff 2012, Till 2009, Tschumi 1996). Traditionally, speaking of architecture is done with an "institutional voice" from *within* the discipline, and as such excluding non-authoritative perspectives (i.e. the multiple voices of the users). As Trefry and Watson (2013, 4) argue, "[i]n architectural education this mode of discourse supports a positivist, or objectively determined, function of architecture in society". This situation induces questions about who has the right to speak for a building–is it the professional architect/researcher or is it the untrained individual "who spent their life living or working in the building, witness to ten thousand sunsets, ten thousand different sounds, ten thousand of chances to touch and smell the place intimately?" (Trefry and Watson 2013, 4). To invite users of the built environment to participate in meaning-making and value formulation, together with trained professionals, might thus call for other methods of assembling such experiences and other means of translation.

Bypassing the "obsession" with the architectural blueprint/drawing and developing other ways to conceive lived experiences could be a first step to reach other, and perhaps deeper, understandings of experiences in relation to use and space (cf. Ballantyne 2004, Cuff 2012, Tschumi 1996). It might also switch the focus from allowing solutions, in turn framed by representational measures, to defining problems. Planning and architecture are often understood in terms of problem-solving, where problems are seen as "a lack" that would disappear with the right solution (Hillier and Abrahams 2013, 24). Instead of considering problems as matters that can ultimately be solved, an alternative conception of problem-solving would take seriously ways of creating spaces, "supporting areas", for negotiating possibilities of various kinds and recognising trade-offs (i.e. a possibility for someone/something is not a possibility for someone/something else).

Let us now travel back and step into Saltsjöbaden Mental Health Centre (SMHC), one of the three outpatient clinics of the Nacka Project, and experience the clinic's performance, its furniture, colours, smells, sounds, patients waiting, people coming and going in and out of rooms, staff moving around, group sessions, medication practices, and so on. The narratives conveyed by staff in documents and interviews, in themselves (re)presentations and translations, and the materiality of the clinic are points of departure for discussing how experiences, activities and materialities of a certain space/time-situated "care architecture" might be understood, conceptualised and perhaps also designed from a relational-material position.

A new clinic for "the new psychiatry"

The Nacka Project was one of the first projects in Sweden to take over total responsibility for mental healthcare in a defined geographical locality. The goal was "to seek and provide a decent and effective alternative to in-patient care" (Berggren and Cullberg 1978, 21), a formulation embedding criticism of in-patient care in general and of mental hospitals in particular, but also incorporating other ways of working with mental health problems. Locating smaller outpatient clinics in the local neighbourhood was seen as a way to avoid institutionalising effects and to achieve normalisation and integration, aiming at preventing people from becoming long-term psychiatric patients and supporting their recovery. The project was imbued with an ethos of de-stigmatising mental health problems and fostering meetings on equal terms among staff and between staff and patients. The staff worked in teams and engaged in therapeutic and preventive work, the former from a social psychiatric and psycho-analytic perspective, the latter at the level of public health and societal planning.

On completion, the Nacka Project became a model for scaling up mental healthcare services to the national level and a well-known example of decentralised Swedish mental healthcare, in particular thanks to substantial media and research coverage at the time (cf. Berggren and Cullberg 1978, Eliasson-Lappalainen 1979, Crafoord 1987) and even today (Cullberg 2007, Jersild 2015). What is less well known, however, is how the spatial configuration of the clinics interacted with usage and users, nor if/how this interaction was related to the Nacka Project's care ideology, encompassing visions and measures of decentralisation. In other words, what did take place (and how) in a pioneering mental health clinic in the 1970s?

Programming visions and preconditions

The care ideology was spatialised at a regional scale by the bureaucratic division of care into defined geographical areas (i.e. sectors), and at local scale by localising smaller outpatient clinics and other care services within neighbourhoods close to where people lived (Berggren and Cullberg 1978). However, the intentions of how exactly to organise and to design outpatient clinics at the scale of individual buildings were not greatly elaborated to any great extent in reports on the Nacka Project. Staff interviews revealed that two teams more or less moved into given premises without really reflecting on their potential advantages or disadvantages, while the third was offered premises designed for storage, with bare concrete walls, neither decorated nor furnished. One staff member, the psychologist Claes, recalled it as "just grey and dark, and there were builders' work lights" (interview[2]). It seemed difficult to imagine this "raw" state becoming something else, but, encouraged by the architect, the staff and managers soon became engaged in a design process, bringing their own experiences from previous workplaces and merging them with visions of how this clinic should perform.

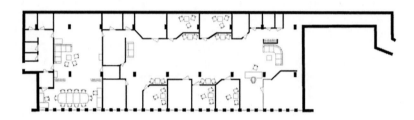

Fig. 7.1. Layout of Saltsjöbaden Mental Health Centre (SMHC). Furnished plan by Arvid Forsberg after the original by Dina Rajs in Spri 1981, 56.

The *Saltsjöbaden Mental Health Centre* opened in 1975 and therapy, counselling and medication work were carried out at the clinic. Staff also did outreach work (e.g. advising social services and the police on mental ill-health). The premises had a rectangular form and windows on only one of the long sides (Fig. 7.1). The limited number of windows promoted a design that allowed light to reach deep into the premises, but resulted in some inner rooms being windowless. To enter the clinic, it was necessary to pass along a narrow corridor, without natural light, which ended in a spacious waiting area. The entrance part of the waiting area was furnished with a noticeboard and a large coat-rack, which, together with a huge curved sofa, divided the entrance area from the waiting area. The reception space was placed in direct connection to the waiting area, the entrance and the sofa. Seven counselling rooms opened directly off the waiting area, without any corridor for distributing movements. The wall was angled towards the counselling rooms, providing seating in shallow alcoves. At the rear of the building was a staff area, a dedicated room where the staff worked together around a large conference table. The walls of the clinic were painted white, on the floor there was a grey wall-to-wall carpet and from the ceiling brown-coloured metal lamps were suspended. The sofa was orange-coloured and the upholstery of the armchairs in the alcoves was striped brown and beige. As a spacing machine (cf. Deleuze and Guattari 2004), elaborating with effects of light, space, sound, colours, materiality and atmosphere (vibrant, calm, quiet, noisy etc.), this architecture made durable a spatial organisation revolving around the waiting area, thus focusing time-space activities such as waiting and passing through.

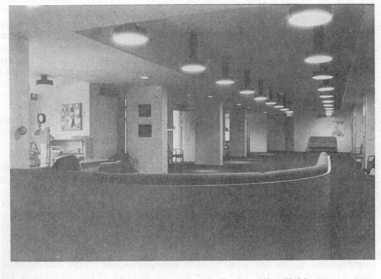

Figure 1.   The Plaza viewed from the Hall

Fig. 7.2. The waiting space, the Plaza, with its spacious floor area, considered by some of the staff interviewed to be the "heart" of the clinic. In this picture it is all empty, and we have to imagine patients coming, waiting, talking, leaving, staff moving back and forth from the staffroom, the receptionist typing, doors opening and closing, all spaced by the large floor area, a smooth atmosphere created by the grey wall-to-wall carpet, white-coloured walls and limited natural light. The orange-coloured sofa-event in the middle acts as a possible contrast to the smooth atmosphere and a central point for emerging activities. Photograph from Szecsödy et al. 1980, 311. Reprinted with permission from Springer.

In the proceedings of a conference in 1980 entitled *Architectural boundaries and their impact on social organisation*, the team leader at SMHC, psychiatrist and psychoanalyst Imre Szecsödy, (re)presented the intentions of the clinic's design. Openness and accessibility to society, as well as establishing common goals and boundaries for staff-patient interactions, were identified as major design objectives for the clinic. They were interpreted architecturally by dividing the premises into four demarcated "territories" (Szecsödy et al. 1980, 309): Hall, Plaza (Fig. 7.2), Cells and Backstage. The alcoves, named Niches (Fig. 7.3), in the waiting room were also considered territory with a distinct function. Spatial setting was viewed as hugely important, in the sense of seeing "individual development in the context of mutual interaction between the person–with his constitutional and psychological endowments–and his physical and social environment" (Szecsödy et al. 1980, 309). The naming of the spaces was therefore a vital event in the re-conceptualising of psychiatric outpatient clinics, as was the spacing of intentions, an event-making "that harbours the possibility of new forms of organising and new political imaginations" (Beyes and Steyaert 2011, 55). The architectural design and the territory naming were projective moves within these original intentions about the mental health centre space, thus influencing (and possibly steering) a new way of working in accordance with the care ideology.

Prevention, or at least the delay, of patient subjectification (or the production of a stigmatising patient identity) was spaced by the design of the waiting area, which was aimed at defusing tension and conveying a feeling of normality, accessibility, openness and meeting on equal terms. The fact of entering behind the sofa and the coat-rack, perhaps looking at the noticeboard, was intended to make it easier for people coming for the first time to leave if they preferred, without being registered or "identified" as a patient.

> People were to enter the Centre into the Hall, from where they could overlook the localities and activities therein. They could sit down, read the papers, look, listen, turn and leave–without being approached by the staff. They were to make their own appeal for help "autonomously". (Szecsödy et al. 1980, 309)

A person who came for the first time was put in contact with a counsellor only after voluntarily approaching the receptionist at the desk in the open area. The first talk with a counsellor took place in the waiting area, in one of the Niches, with no coercion or demands. When the person's problem was defined as psychiatric (it could have been social, economic or legal), registration took place, whereby this person was transferred/spaced to the status of patient and then invited into the counselling room as a registered patient together with the counsellor. The patient subjectivity emerged here, in line with the formulation by Jones, McLean, and Quattrone (2004, 724), through "the creation and assemblages of Spacing(s), Timing(s) and Acting(s), i.e. various actions that endeavour to make order". A certain rhythm of openings and closings, what might be termed the *space-acts* inherent in entering the room and closing the door, thus made an ordering of patient/counsellor subjectivities possible.

> In the beginning much openness and little seclusion was offered. As involvement between clients and staff deepened, the higher were the walls

of intimacy and confidentiality raised around them. At the same time it was emphasized that clients and staff would meet on "neutral territory" with shared responsibility all the time. (Szecsödy et al. 1980, 313)

This "psychiatric triage" was not only supposed to delay the application of a psychiatric patient identity, but was also an event-making serving to de-stigmatise mental health problems. The event of passing between the receptionist's desk and the sofa was in this respect an important spacing of change. The help-seeking person literally had to move through this physical space, thereby entering a process of transforming from anonymous person to registered patient. When walking down this passage, a transitory move was enacted and a change of subjectification took place, from unknown to known, from private person to patient, a "turn-around" of doing, thinking and becoming which was entangled with and enacted by materialities (sofa, desk, coat-rack, registration forms etc.), the spatial layout, body movement and talk (cf. Anderson and Harrison 2010a).

The counselling rooms were not personalised. When a staff member needed a counselling room, they simply took any one available. These rooms were all furnished similarly, with armchairs positioned around a coffee table "with the same high quality of Scandinavian type furniture" (Szecsödy et al. 1980, 313). There was a therapeutic idea behind these non-personalised rooms, since they were intended to be a neutral "playground" (cf. Winnicott 2003) for staff-patient interaction, but they were also a measure to foster a non-hierarchical culture within the team. Szecsödy claimed in the interview that counselling roles were not predefined in a non-personalised room, thus providing potential to establish a more equal counsellor-patient relationship. A room already marked in advance by the personality of the counsellor was believed to hamper such relationship building. The event of booking a room for each session, in tandem with the design of the space, thus made possible the "playground". What was programmed was a certain "setting", but one not apprehended as external to the taking-place in the room. Rather, the interior design (similar sparse furniture and discreet colours) and actual organisation of the non-personalised rooms and the counselling event enacted a "neutral space", one which made possible situated material and immaterial relations and durations (Latham and McCormack 2004) for as long as the therapeutic session took place. These non-directed encounters were intended to open up opportunities for alternative events and spacings in every new session (i.e. "the playground" and "the play").

The staffroom, the Backstage, was also an important site for spacing care ideologies and facilitating the event-making of a non-hierarchical staff organisation. No patients were allowed here. The staff worked together in this space, sharing a large conference table. The rationale underpinning the idea of a common work space was that staff members should learn and support from each other, and thereby develop a common ideology (Szecsödy et al. 1980). Daily conferences were held where staff shared information and discussed "emergency calls during the night, new patients, planning of therapies, progress of ongoing therapies. Information was also shared about mental health consultations done in the area as other types of co-operative and preventive activities within the community" (Szecsödy et al. 1980, 313). Administrative staff meetings, supervisory and theoretical seminars took place, as well as the ongoing doings of paperwork, dictations and telephone calls. The Backstage was a spacing of "multiple trajectories" (Beyes and Steyaert 2011, 53); and, as we shall see in the next section, learning certainly occurred, but maybe not in quite such smooth way as described by the team leader Szecsödy.

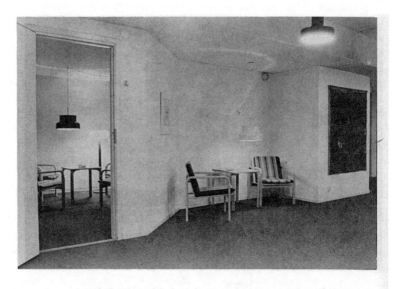

Figure 3.   A Niche with entrance and view into an office, i.e. Cell

Fig. 7.3. A niche with its chairs and table, one of several seating opportunities of the waiting space. To the left, there is a view into the counselling room, with similar chairs, table and lamp as in the Niches and similar white walls and grey carpet. All counselling rooms had similar interior design to make possible the neutral counselling event open to situated relational processes. Photograph from Szecsödy et al. 1980, 312. Reprinted with permission from Springer.

What is striking in the conveyed account is that one important "actor" has largely been omitted, namely the spatial preconditions, the "raw" space, of the former storage facility. What is not observed is its impact on the spatial organisation and design of the clinic's premises. Space is mentioned quite a lot in the accounts, but as a fixed space, a background or a setting for intended activities. However, in interviews with the staff engaged in the design process of the premises (cf. Högström, 2012), the preconditions, the "raw" state, emerge as more influential in organising and designing the clinic than how they are presented by the team leader and in the conference proceedings (Szecsödy et al. 1980). For example, the large waiting space without a corridor (the Plaza), the non-personalised counselling rooms (the Cells) and the common staffroom (the Backstage) were probably not directly transmitted from care-ideological considerations into spatial configurations. Rather, *spacing* in its "raw" state seems to have been just as important for organising and designing processes as were care-ideological visions. Materiality and immateriality are not external to each other, but are co-constitutive and intertwined (Latham and McCormack 2004), which in this design process emerged as non-linear entanglements of material preconditions, care-ideological statements and staff members' previous (spacing) experiences. The material/spatial conditions largely consisted of a limited amount of natural light, as the space had windows on only one of the long sides, which marked the spatial organisation of SMHC. In the accounts conveyed here by Szecsödy (interview) and Szecsödy et al. (1980), SMHC is nonetheless still (re)presented more or less as a fixed space of "brute matter" (cf. Latham and McCormack 2004, 705), a mere setting, trusted to make place for activities but where interference, i.e. blurring/merging/give-and-take of "spacing-timing-acting" (Jones, McLean, and Quattrone 2004), was not recognised.

Spacing events of care in the everyday

How did the Nacka Project's staff recollect SMHC? Did their opinions of "good therapeutic practice" change as the everyday practice took place? According to staff interviews, having worked at SMHC was still a living memory of love and criticism and many of the accounts revolved around the waiting area, the Plaza. The waiting area, considered the heart of the clinic, was spaced in terms of: (1) the many seating possibilities when waiting; (2) the possibility for the receptionist to approach and socialise with patients and visitors in a welcoming manner, while still keeping an eye on the situation; (3) a place for the first encounter with a therapist; and (4) a device for distribution of movements. Marianne, a counsellor, reported that the sofa ("an embracement", as the psychologist Claes said) actually did facilitate contact between patients:

> Sometimes patients sat down [on the sofa] leaving an obvious distance between each other. On another occasion there were two patients who knew each other; they had tried to commit suicide and come back. They started talking to each other.

Nursing assistant Peter claimed that the spacious waiting area was ingenious, as "people who were restless could move around without being too conspicuous". Nurse Marie was more critical, claiming that the openness did not cater well enough for patient protection and anonymity. Counsellor Marianne regarded the Plaza as encouraging "doings of crazy things", and she remembered patients at times doing handstands. She also recalled walking towards the sofa with feelings of being seen, hearing patients commenting "You look so tired!", "Did you get this or that pill?" or "Did you take the green pill, you don't seem awake yet!". On entering the Plaza from Backstage, staff were put on stage, a "cat-walk" enabled by patients, the sofa and the distance from Backstage door and the sofa, leading to a reversal of the traditional staff-patient hierarchy. These different events enacted spacings, as well as spacing enacting events (e.g. encounters between individuals in the sofa, the ability to hear everything in the room, introducing unexpected bodily movements in a space usually conceived as one for "doing-nothing-but waiting", enacting gazes of seeing and being seen).

The waiting area was a spacing where events happened, a place of "mediation, negotiation, openings and closings" (Jones, McLean, and Quattrone 2004, 724), intimately related to practices taking place in rhythms depending on how many people were there at a certain time, the quality of daylight (sunny, cloudy, rainy) reaching into the premises, the amount of doors being opened or closed, and the number of people talking or walking around. According to statements in staff interviews, the generosity of the waiting area assisted in staff security, through the fact that absence of pressure on patients tended to discourage violent situations. Such an "opening" led to patients rarely becoming violent, while another "opening" was the "relaxed" design of the reception and the friendly way of meeting patients supported by the design. This matter is exemplified by a "closing" reported by receptionist Gertrud: "after going through the horrible dark and cold corridor, it was probably good to see a human there". Gertrud's memories of the waiting area, though, are not entirely positive. Instead of the Plaza, she called the space "the Hangar", referring to its sparse furnishing and white and grey colours, and perhaps to spacing-timings (Jones, McLean, and Quattrone 2004) when it was empty of people. Peter, the nursing assistant, recalled that patients respected not being allowed into the staffroom. The door was placed at the back of the waiting space, at the side of the double wall and less visible from the sofa and other seatings. As such, boundaries were marked by spatial means and no locks were needed. However, on a few occasions patients reportedly did not respect this boundary and entered the staffroom, but, according to Peter, these cases were entirely diagnostic: "they were completely mad". Events such as handstands, walking back and forth, chatting and gazing all encompassed mediations and negotiations of boundaries, as well as fluid relations between materialities, people, affects, objects and movements (cf. Anderson and Harrison 2010a). Boundaries on what to do and not to do were negotiated constantly, but when what was the only really strict border of the clinic (i.e. the door to Backstage) was transgressed, it was by persons whose borders of reality had arguably already been transgressed.

Hierarchy was a recurring issue during the clinic's lifetime and the Backstage spaced many of these events (cf. Eliasson-Lappalainen 1979). Closing off patients opened it up for other openings. The experiences of Backstage differed, as some staff considered it a non-hierarchical spacing of knowledge transfer and cooperation, while others pointed out a lack of integrity and difficulties in concentrating. For example, the horizontal staff organisation was challenged from the very start by a specific space-act. When the team moved in, according to the psychologist Claes, the team leader Szecsödy, who had promoted the collective model, took one of the counselling rooms as his personal office. He claimed that, as head of unit, he needed a special room to receive guests. By "spacing" such a hierarchical event, fundamental ideals were seemingly violated, which had consequences because the team members responded to Szecsödy's space-act with indignation and forced him back into the Backstage area to work there alongside all of the other staff. "We were so strong. He had no choice", Claes reported. Even so, unlike the staff who worked together at the conference table, Szecsödy put his typewriter on top of a wheeled cabinet in one corner, occupying that zone for himself; and as such, he enacted superiority within the material possibilities that remained available to him. The spacing taking place by Szecsödy's appropriation of the corner was not only an event of personalising work-places, but also an event of surveillance: "[t]he office in the corner helped to do leadership work adequately, to have a general overview of the activities of the staff, to aid and control the staff" (Szecsödy et al. 1980, 314). This quote is contradictory to the idea of the common workplace as a spacing of cooperation and learning. The team leader put himself outside of the dynamic and fluid events around the conference table, and instead he spaced hierarchy and surveillance.

Nursing assistant Peter recalled that the period of acclimatisation was shorter than in other places where he had worked, because "the work was visible all the time". The Backstage design encouraged a working atmosphere imbued with flexibility and fellowship, but this collective idea also demanded a high degree of personal self-control among the staff members. According to the interviews, the people around the table had to talk in a low voice, keep papers and other objects in order, and accept that someone might have taken the chair they wanted. This state of being proved to be difficult to uphold in the long run. Tensions developed within the team and unexpected, maybe undesirable events took place, such as people choosing to work by themselves in vacant counselling rooms. The common workspace was thus not entirely appreciated by all staff at all times. Nurse Marie complained in interview that, while the team leader sat in his corner:

> We others drifted around. I myself sat in the cloakroom while dictating. One had everything in a notebook and on the conference table. If you left to see a patient, on returning someone might have made a mess out of everything. Once I found a big coffee-ring on one of my case books.

Negotiations of ordering slowly changed the flexibility of Backstage towards a more fixed space with clear functions. Places around the table became more or less permanently occupied by staff members. The initial fluid spacing seemed difficult to cope with for many staff members. When the team leader Szecsödy quit after three years, Marie, the nurse, managed to get left-over desks and telephones (ironically from the negative other of "the new psychiatry", the old asylum, which was about to close down). The main table was replaced by personal workplaces with telephones, although, as Marie commented, the awkwardness of working together in one large room remained:

> Some colleagues might be talking about a movie they had seen while I had a patient on the phone saying "I just wanted to say that I am going to commit suicide and I have filled the bathtub with water".

The mediation of experiences was emphasised further when a re-organisation took place shortly after Marie's instalment of personal desks. Another team moved to SMHC and contested the spatial organisation immediately. The common work-space and the non-personalised counselling rooms were the main target of their criticism, dismissed as non-workable spacings. Claes, the psychologist, recalled:

> They couldn't understand how we could work like this .... [They criticised] everything from, "I couldn't imagine not having a room of my own", which

we couldn't understand, "you only have to book", to talking about patients getting hurt by being in different rooms on every occasion.

When different practices meet and mould, changes and conflicts emerge. The attention of the new team members was on the spatial configuration as a separate entity (absolute space), external to spacings of work organisation, care ideology and spatial preconditions (the "raw" state), mediated and negotiated on everyday practice basis. Contestations of the associated spacings and events became a challenging obstacle, fuelling events of mistrust and discontent. Even though it was more than thirty years ago, Peter, a nursing assistant at the time, remembers his sad feeling when the team eventually left SMHC:

> I remember how sad I thought it was. Now it [the new premises] looked like any hospital corridor anywhere in Sweden. The special time was over.

How this "special time", with these experiences, spacings and events that took place, became translated into guidelines for outpatient clinics of the future is discussed in the next section.

Guidelining the future–a solution to what problem?

As mentioned, much attention was paid to the Nacka Project at the time, and it was in this context that *the Swedish Health and Social Care Institute for Planning and Rationalisation* (SPRI) decided to evaluate the "new psychiatry". SPRI, which existed between 1968 and 2000, conducted research and development work and acted as the advisory body to the healthcare business (SPRI 1985). One of its tasks was to develop solutions for care facilities, it being noted that the transition of psychiatric care from mental hospitals to community care created a need for rethinking facility design. The report series *Psychiatry in Transition* (1977-1986) aimed at scrutinising such needs, and two of the reports in the series (SPRI 1983, 1981) had the objective of formulating design recommendations for new psychiatric outpatient care facilities. The Nacka Project's mental health centres, especially SMHC, were used as objects in the evaluation, as well as precedents for recommendations. Room categories, areas and desirable links between functional units were exemplified in the SPRI reports with the help of observations, environmental analysis, interviews and questionnaires. The reports tried to find answers to problems of localisation (separate outpatient clinics or inside hospitals), accessibility (housing areas or shopping centres), standards (hospital standards) and whether forms of cooperation influenced the design. They were illustrated by interior photographs, diagrams showing links between rooms, recommended measures and sketches showing suggestions for furniture and furnishings. Locations and spatial organisations were also represented in images and blueprints. Regarding the design of physical environments, the report stated that psychiatric outpatient clinics should have "a simple and modest atmosphere" (SPRI 1983, 38). An open and light character was to be achieved by short corridors and ample daylight, and it was considered important not to reproduce an hospital-like atmosphere.

SMHC was described as interesting in terms of spatial layout, practicality and "without institutional or hospital atmosphere" (SPRI 1981, 85), but the one-sided natural light and the large waiting room were seen as disadvantages. No account was taken of how such a large waiting area could contribute something valuable, in contrast to what emerged during staff interviews. The way of (re)presenting the spacings of SMHC here seemed "to invoke a realm of reassuringly tangible or graspable objects" (Latham and McCormack 2004, 704). The focus was on the objects as measurable realities, without taking into account the complex relations "held together and animated by processes excessive of form and position" (705). The findings and analysis made by SPRI were marked by an apparently absolute space conceptualisation, as a "deductive reasoning of a homogeneous voice" (Trefry and Watson 2013, 4), implying that it is possible to define general measures on what a "good" clinic ought to be.

According to SPRI guidelines, the architectural design should give the clinic an "inviting and special character" (SPRI 1983, 38) and the interior as a whole should be "functional and nice" (39). Value-laden adjectives were used to define objectives for the clinic's design, in a way of "mastering conditions and providing correct answers" (Trefry and Watson 2013, 4).

> The interior should be designed to give the visitor a "homely" feeling and the environment should facilitate a relaxed and trustful contact between visitor and therapist. Furnishing should be simple and comfortable and consist of few types of furniture of good quality. (SPRI 1983, 38)

The waiting space at SMHC was described by SPRI as an example worth noting–in terms of the "step-by-step" contact (i.e. "psychiatric triage") and the choice of seating. Parts of the corridor in front of the counselling rooms could in some cases also be used as a waiting area. The corridor should in that case be either wider or be designed with niches for smaller waiting areas. The first contact between therapist and patient could be made in these smaller waiting units. One solution with the "step-by-step contact" has been completed in Nacka in SMHC's premises. Waiting patients should have a certain choice in where they want to sit, so that they can either choose the vicinity of other patients in a sofa, at a round table or privacy in smaller waiting areas.

This account leaves out the objectives for the spatial and furnishing arrangements. To a great extent, only solutions are presented, thus in effect defining the problems in retrospect (Hillier and Abrahams 2013). For example, the corridor is taken for granted, but adjusted in width to the activities proposed; the sectioned sofa is a functional answer to questions of room size and shape; and it is implied that the patients create dirt and. have difficulties with mobility. More ambiguity is shown, however, regarding the staffroom and counselling rooms

> How could [a common staffroom] be designed, and what would it mean to work in [such a room]? A certain scepticism to new ways of working is natural. People are most afraid of losing their territory and privacy. The employees should decide for themselves whether they want to work in a personalised room, or if the advantages of a common staffroom outweigh these. (SPRI 1983, 22)

There is a reluctance to come up with solutions in a matter defined here as personal. In this ordering process, complex and entangled issues of spacings and events, the "relational-material account of 'the social'" (Anderson and Harrison 2010a, 13), are not given attention. Instead, the issue of the staffroom is compartmentalised as a question of individual choice. Thus, although approaches to work organisation are mentioned in this quote, the overall impression is that recommendations are formulated and visualised in a manner based on how and what to furnish. This focus leaves out the multi-faceted experiences revealed in interviews and bypasses spacings and events taking place when architecture, operation and users come together. (Re)presentation is differentiation and transformation (Doel 2010), not direct transmission of facts. As such, the reports act as *presentations* that certainly enact SMHC as things and activities, as transmission of facts. If we were to use conventional means of representing space (i.e. architectural blueprints), these would show SMHC merely as a fragmented spacing; as non-contextualised pockets of arrangements of objects (furniture). Overall, the reports are detached from both user experiences and programmatic accounts. The latter aimed at a projective entanglement of spatial configuration, care ideology and work organisation in order to meet visions of "the new psychiatry", while the former told different stories about everyday practices of care and transient/fluid/differential spacing and events.

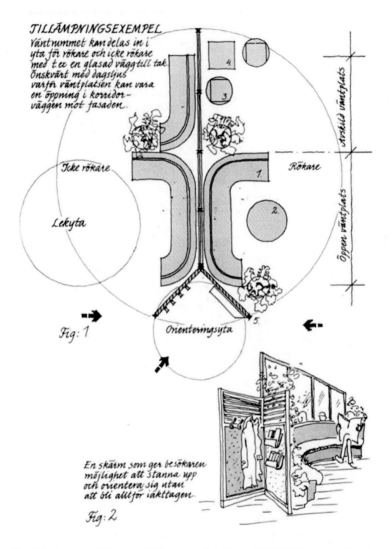

Fig. 7.4. An excerpt from a SPRI report showing, with SMHC as precedent, how a waiting area of an outpatient clinic for the "new psychiatry" could be furnished. 1) A layout with sofas divided by a screen to provide privacy and to divide smokers from non-smokers. On the non-smoking side, there is a space marked "play area", presupposing children coming to the clinic. 2) A layout with the screen also acted as a notice board. Drawing by Uno Lindh & Eva Linnman, Svenska rum, in SPRI 1983, 14.

Thus, the situated practices of SMHC were largely translated into measurable objects set in absolute space, and as such possible to represent within "[a] supposed neutrality of metric space" (Till 2009, 122) and as a solution to problems not clearly defined (cf. Hillier and Abrahams 2013).

Reflections

In this chapter, I have highlighted issues of programming, experiencing and guide-lining spaces based on an analysis of the *Saltsjöbaden Mental Health Centre* (SMHC). While SMHC only lasted for a couple of years in the late-1970s at the particular geographical location described in this chapter, it has left immaterial and material accounts, in terms of: (1) situated experiences of work organisation, management, presumptions, personal backgrounds, group dynamics, hopes and disappointments; (2) programming for intentional experiences; (3) guidelining recommendations for future design of outpatient clinics; and (4) material preconditions framing the design and organisation of the clinic (i.e. the "raw" state of the premises before re-design). Architecture, understood as events and spacings, opens up an apprehension of the braided relations between immaterialities, materialities, emergences and durations (cf. Latham and McCormack 2004, Jones, McLean, and Quattrone 2004, Beyes and Steyaert 2011).

   If architecture is understood as events and spacings, is it possible to (re)present such multiple experiences without closing off potentials and possibilities? Or, as Anderson and Harrison (2010a, 22) put it: "[h]ow ... to relate to the future without capturing it and neutralising it before it happens?". This is likely to be in a question of knowledge, concerning the grounds on which spac*ings* are conceived and how this conception frames (re)presentation. From an architectural practice point of view, adopting a non-representational understanding of space as "doings" and "differentials" (i.e. as events and spacings) challenges certain fundamentals of practice–the supposed generative work of design, as emerging through representational means (i.e. sketches, blueprints, models). However, it is not only generative but also prescriptive, and herein may lie the most crucial challenge for rethinking architecture and its representational legacy. Architecture is also, beside its experiential and emerging spacings, an assemblage of material components. In order to accomplish such a composition (i.e. in order to build), prescriptions are needed, even if this representation is carried out solely by talking and pointing at the construction site without any blueprints drawn up by building consultants. Projection of visions for the future which represent intentions stemming from lived experiences–and which acknowledge emergent potentialities and possibilities, taking seriously spacing and events–

calls for a rethinking of architectural practice methodologies and, in particular, an altered conception of writing guidelines (e.g. why, what and how to (re)present conditions for the future): "[r]ather than attempt to lay out a prescription for encounters, perhaps it is better to offer some tactical suggestions" (Dewsbury et al. 2002, 439). Promoting a more open-ended way of working with recommendations for the future would be to displace "solutions" to provisional principles and let in other voices than only "the institutional voice" (Trefry and Watson 2013, 4). Nothing is ever completely solved, since "[w]hatever we decide to do, we could always have done something else" (Hillier and Abrahams 2013, 24). As such, any articulation (guidelines, drawing, model etc.) is stable only for a short moment of time before the spacing of events continues. This way of thinking entails broader (re)presentational repertoires for architects and other spatial agents working in the care industry, particularly when translating immaterialities and materialities into guidelines for future car*ing* architectures.

Notes

[1] During the period 1967-1995, Swedish mental healthcare underwent a complete re-organisation, starting with county councils taking over responsibility for mental healthcare from the state. Mental hospitals were slowly phased out and replaced with community care. Under the Psychiatry Reform of 1995, decentralisation took one step further as local councils took charge of housing and employment for people with long-term mental ill-health.
[2] Unless otherwise noted, all translations of interview quotes are my own.

COMMENTARY IV

FROM CARING ARCHITECTURE TO THE ARCHITECTURE OF CARE

ALBENA YANEVA

The growing influence of the pragmatist philosophy has gradually changed the way we think of our built environment and has shifted the focus from architecture as meaning to architecture as process and becoming, from the lives of those who inhabit the cities to the life of buildings and other material entities. The book *Caring Architecture* draws on a relational perspective that takes inspiration from recent development in geography and science studies. Architecture became a new terrain for STS-trained anthropologists as early as 2000, who following a programmatic article of Michel Callon (1996), engaged in tracing design in the making (Houdart 2008, Houdart and Minato 2009, Loukissas 2012, Yaneva 2009a, 2005). Drawing on the way STS engaged in analysis of science in the making and the scientific practices of visualization (Lynch 1985, 1993, Lynch and Edgerton 1988, Lynch and Woolgar 1990, Latour 2000, Pickering 1992, Galison 1997) the new ethnographies of architecture focused on accounting the hands-on process of architectural experimentation and "interpretation" as an art situated within the performance of design practice. These studies contributed to a better understanding of the visualization practices, distributed thinking, instruments, communication, material culture, and design environment. Whilst STS-informed research focused on architecture as embedded in complex networks of design practice, geographers provided interpretations of architecture as embedded in the practice of inhabitation, dwelling within and interacting with the "living body" of a building or a performative urban environment. Rather than profiling architects and their "tribes" as professional groups, anthropologists traced the materialization of design operations and the socio-material complexity of design outlining the routines, actions and transactions of all participants in design in compound spatial settings.

Both groups of scholars shared the assumption that architecture cannot be reduced to a static frame of symbolic meaning (Latour and Yaneva 2008); that a deeper understanding of architecture can be gained by studying ordinary unfolding courses of action in design, use, inhabitation, maintenance, reuse and contestation. In their articulation of a mode of processual inquiry into the life of buildings, geographers tackled the ways in which space, performance and event are shaped in the process of use, inhabitation, and evaluation of buildings and urban spaces. The themes tackled included: the work of maintenance (Graham and Thrift 2007), the interactions of bodies and everyday practices in designed urban environments (Degen, Rose, and Basdas 2010), the mundane "life of buildings" that appeared in their accounts as being reminiscent to "living bodies" (Jacobs, Cairns, and Strebel 2007, Strebel 2011), and "practising architectures" (Jacobs and Merriman 2011). In this work geographers took much inspiration from STS (and in particular from the work of Bruno Latour), which, transformed by the influence of socio-cultural anthropology, resulted in extensive ethnographic studies of scientific and technological processes. A number of typologies have been studied from an Actor-Network-Theory-inspired relational perspective: museums, housing complexes, towers, megaprojects. Yet, little is known about the typology of caring architecture.

Buildings serve both as active agents in the transformation of patients and their identity and as a living evidence for these changes. At the same time, architects, planners, interior designers think about how patients and caregivers use and inhabit these spaces, how they move through these facilities and how the material arrangements enhance practices of medicalization, hospitalisation and recovery. The structure and materiality of spaces, surfaces and spatial transitions reflect the funding realities and socio-economic climates; yet, they have an agency on their own. Following how exactly patients and caregivers use these buildings (according to architect expectations or by misusing the buildings; by following the script of the buildings or by adapting and re-appropriating space according to their needs), one can witness how architecture acts as a guiding, daily reminder to patients, medical practitioners and caregivers of who they are and where they stand. By exposing the adjacency and distance between different groups of patients and caregivers, between ready-made treatment and experimentation, the built world helps define how care professionals see themselves. And this is one of the key messages of this book.

The volume attempts to overcome architectural determinism from one side (architecture determinative of the medical and nursing treatment /care conducted inside) and architectural indifference, on the other (architecture irrelevant to the modalities of care contained within its walls). Enticing the readers to witness the socio-material practices of care giving facilitated by various spatio-material arrangements and the design of hospital and psychiatry buildings, asylums, and nursing homes, the book invites us to explore how buildings of care literally and figuratively configure the practices and identities of patients and caregivers as well as the very field of care giving. Conversely, we witness how care giving and medicalization inform us about the shifting practices of architects and interior designers.

Design and space matter in care giving. Material and spatial transformations do have an impact on the efficiency of care. The book tells us *how* and expands on the specific features of buildings and material arrangements that better cater for the needs of caring architecture. For instance, most care providing buildings today contain adaptable and flexible spaces that evolve over time: the contemporary care giving architecture has more spatial and mechanical flexibility and this is particularly significant today for accommodating dynamic change inside, change that involves flexible activities, processes and technologies. Flexibility is essential to the fast-changing world of care giving and the need for spatial adaptability to the specific dispositive of care and the importance to update the spatial and technological equipment.

In addition to the spatial distribution, it is important to consider the use of materials in care buildings and the maintenance strategies they imply. The choice between concrete, teak, lead, glass, and special steel is not an innocent one. To enhance further the human element in a highly technical medical environment, natural materials such as oak can be chosen for wainscoting, doors, furniture, and casework. Daylight is considered as crucial for the patients' well-being, and this leads architects to choose glass over other materials. All these choices are important as they facilitate different types of care for patients. Sometimes the choices made by the architect might not be the choices of patients and caregivers. For instance, if an architect considers natural light and space as the most important ingredients of good caring architecture, these might not be the key features for good caring environments for the users; natural light might be good for living rooms and leisure spaces in a caring home, but it might not be suitable for medical environments where it can hamper the success of experiments and interact with chemicals in an unpredictable way.

Moreover, the design of individual and collective space is also a question of careful political choice. The growing importance of atria and lounge spaces in hospital today is crucial; they bring people together and help to avoid segregation among patients whose treatment usually demands isolated and controlled environments. A caring building is never a stable container that frames the practices of caregivers and patients. Its spaces vary according to the different modalities of action of patients and caregivers in a way that we have a multitude of different spaces: closed, quiet spaces for individual patients; open, public spaces for spontaneous activities and leisure activates outside the highly specialised medical spaces; research space that also encourage the continuous exchange of information between medical specialists; generous circulation spaces such as staircase or other lounge spaces that invites exchanges between and among floors as people constantly pass each other and relate their patient or care giving experiences; offices grouped in clusters or in separate spaces reinforcing the sense of community among different types of practitioners and patients or segregating them even more; spaces for spontaneous interactions and gatherings. Through the sharing of spaces, resources and facilities, architects can effectively promote the sharing of care experience and the companionate human dialogue among patients.

Caring architecture is a specialized building type. Yet, architecture is not fundamentally about places, it's principally about people doing things *enabled* and *facilitated* by space. The success of caring architecture would depend on the genuine collaboration between the medical and psychology practitioners and the architects of care giving buildings (hospitals, asylums, nursing homes). How do we design buildings that do not simply accomplish a basic programme, but do something more: i.e. facilitate people interacting with each other so that cured patient can share experience with others, make them feel more comfortable, more independent? Good caring buildings cannot be constructed without any knowledge about the practices they are supposed to house; that is another important message of the book. Architects and designers should pay close attention to the needs of patients and caregivers to design places where people interact and have both structured and informal contact.

In addition, the design of care buildings holds an important political question–what power is given to patients to configure and reconfigure the care spaces as they see fit. What type of care politics is embedded in the way walls and doors divide or puts patients and caregivers together? How do hospitals, nursing homes, asylums, and other care providing facilities procedurally and metaphorically structure the practices of architects and designers? Equally, what can caring architecture tell us about the changing nature of care giving?

The book posits an important question: What is care? How do space and materiality matter in the complex socio-material process of care giving? How do different types of caring architecture overcome the duality between subject and object, meaning and materiality? How then does person-centred care appear in a context of spatio-material processes? As is asked in the Introduction: is person-centred care a relevant notion after all? Care is understood in this book as something that cannot be provided by a sudden gesture of subject-object transformation; care, or the process of caring implies the gradual transformation of a whole *dispositif* (setting) that slowly and painstakingly transforms objects into subjects and subjects into objects. Taking care implies a regime of agency that would suppose that many spatial arrangements and actors gradually transform in a network in a way that the less autonomous and independent objects will be rendered human, autonomous.

Thus the architectural setting of care giving should be designed in a way that it can provide conditions for gaining increasingly degrees of autonomy and liberty. In other words, the book explores what sits between the two extremities: neglect and abandon for patients, on one hand, and autonomous subjective agency, on the other. Architectural environments of hospitals, nursing houses, asylums are seen here as providing facilities that assist the slow modifications of subjects and objects captured in complex spatial medical/caring settings: patients, caring personnel, material arrangements substances, medical devices, technologies and equipment, material arrangements. Caring architecture tackles the spatial complexity of care as an ensemble of all the networked efforts of care giving that take place between independence and dependence, objectivity and subjectivity.

Caring architecture implies a type of architecture that helps the transformation of a particular subject, typically a sick person, a troubled youngster or an aged adult in need of regular nursing, into a patent of care. Yet, architecture does not provide containers for caring programmes; it rather shapes a subtle networked setting that makes possible the process of caring to be efficient. The book compels us to overcome the duality between the presence of an active subject providing and delivering care and a passive object, receiving care. With the help of architecture, the subject receiving care is slowly and gradually turned into a subject endowed with more degrees of autonomy. Care giving facilitates the many different trials, experiments, and adjustments of objects and subjects; it is the architectural setting that provides the conditions for many objects to pass from activity to passivity and back. The mediation of patient' treatment–facilitated by technologies, equipment, medical professionals, materials and spaces–makes possible the action to pass from one state to another. The complex spatial networks of the caring regime offer conditions for patients to gain more autonomy, more degrees of subjectivity and liberty and to get transformed into subjects, more performing, more alive, cured. For this to happen, we need a network of caring actors, instruments, devices, settings and other objects to be assembled in the process of care giving. The networks of care giving are complex; their architecture deserves careful treatment. The book demonstrates convincingly how important is this transition: from *caring architecture* to the *care for architecture*.

CONTRIBUTORS

Morgan Andersson is an architect and holds a PhD in Architecture from Chalmers University of Technology, where he is currently a guest researcher at the Centre of Healthcare Architecture. His main focus is housing for an ageing population, especially aspects of housing and care. Previously, he has studied building projects in Swedish forensic psychiatry.

Erling Björgvinsson is a Professor of Design at The Academy of Design and Crafts, University of Gothenburg. He researches on participatory politics in design and art. Among other things, in the research project *Placebo*, he studies how patient perspectives on hospital architecture can inform spatial issues in hospitals.

Martin Gren is Associate Professor at the Linnaeus University. He has had a longstanding interest in "geographiology" with a focus on how the relations between humans and the Earth are depicted and enacted in social thought-and-practice. His most recent work is the co-edited book *Tourism and Anthropocene* (Routledge, 2016).

Ebba Högström is Senior Lecturer in Urban Studies at Blekinge Institute of Technology and Director of the Master Programme in Urban Planning. She has a PhD in Planning and Decision Analysis from KTH, Stockholm and a long experience from architectural practice. Her research interests concern institutions, planning and architecture in a socio-material perspective with a special interest in asylum and mental health spaces.

Ingunn Moser is Professor of Sociology and Social Studies of Science and Technology at Diakonhjemmet University College in Oslo. Her research centres on relations between subjectivity, embodiment, materiality and knowledge. These theoretical interests are being explored in empirical fields ranging from disability to care for the elderly and dementia care in particular.

Catharina Nord is Associate Professor at Spatial Planning at Blekinge Institute of Technology. She has a long experience in research about ageing and architecture. Currently, she is working on architectural space and care practice in assisted living facilities. She explores these institutional buildings mainly with the support of theories about relational space, assemblage theory and actor-network theory.

Gunnar Olsson is currently Professor Emeritus at the University of Uppsala. For a lifetime he has been exploring the no-man's land between categories, all in search of the invisible Palace of Power (itself invisible), its imagined blueprint a multidimensional chiasm of identity and difference, picture and story, one and many, ontology and epistemology. His latest book is *Abysmal: A Critic of Cartographic Reason* (University of Chicago Press, 2007).

Chris Philo is Professor of Geography in the School of Geographical & Earth Sciences, University of Glasgow. His research centres on what could be termed *the historical geography of the "mad-business"* in England and Wales. He also works on a wide range of asylum-related topics, including attention to: animals, "madness" and asylums; patient artwork and physician analyses, linking with psychoanalytic and psychotherapeutic geographies.

Kim Ross holds a PhD in Human Geography from the School of Geographical & Earth Sciences, University of Glasgow. Her research looks into the emergence and development of the later "Asylum Age" in nineteenth century Scotland, looking specifically at district asylums from 1857 to 1913. She is currently a secondary school Geography teacher in Scotland.

Gunnar Sandin is Associate Professor in Architecture at Lund University. His research concerns site specificity in a political and aesthetic perspective, as reflected for instance in the article "Democracy on the margin" in *Architectural Theory Review*. He is currently leading the research project *The Evolutionary Periphery*, which explores issues of land use.

Susanne Severinsson is Associate Professor in Pedagogic Practices, a trained social worker with a PhD in Educational Science. Recent work concern education for students in juvenile foster care and how pedagogical practices construct and reconstruct the teenagers and vice versa. Her current activities include lecturing and research in special education and social work at Linköping University.

Albena Yaneva is Professor of Architectural Theory and Director of Manchester Research Centre at the University of Manchester. She has published extensively in the field of anthropology of art and architecture, spanning the disciplinary boundaries of architectural theory, sociology, science studies and political philosophy. Her current work centres on politics of architecture and the practices of archiving in the arts.

REFERENCE LIST

Primary Sources Chapter Four

Ayr District Board Annual Report. 1872. Second Annual Report of the Ayr District Asylum. Ayr: Printed at the Ayr Advertiser Office. Centre for Archive and Information Services, Dundee, THB 30/6/1/8.

Ayr Hospital Minute Book. 1879. Ayrshire District Lunacy Board. Unpublished. Ayr Archives, AA17/4/2.

Glasgow District Board Annual Report. 1898. First Report of the City of Glasgow District Lunacy Board with the Medical Superintendent's Report, together with Reports by her Majesty's Commissioners in Lunacy, and an Abstract of the Treasurer's Accounts. Glasgow: printed by N. Adshead & Son, 11 and 92 Union Street. NHS Greater Glasgow and Clyde Archives, HB1/6/1.

Haddington Asylum Patient Book. 1868. Unpublished hand-written entries by General Commissioners in Lunacy. Lothian Health Board Archives, LHB47/2/1/1.

Free Press. 1904. Kingseat Asylum–Report by the Commissioners in Lunacy–Congratulations to District Board. October 24th. NHS Grampian Archives, GRHB 8/6/2.

Evening Gazette. 1906. New Treatment for the Insane–No Strait Jackets and Dark Cells. June 6th. NHS Grampian Archives, GRHB 8/6/2.

Tenth Annual Report of the Ayr District Asylum. 1880. Ayr: Printed at the Ayr Advertiser Office. Ayr Archives, THB 30/6/1/8. Ayr District Board Minute Book 1880.

SCL. 1862. Fourth Annual Report of the General Board of Commissioners in Lunacy for Scotland. Paper Number: 2974, Volume/page: XXIII.255, CH Microfiche Number: 68.147-150:1-255.

SCL. 1864. Sixth Annual Report of the General Board of Commissioners in Lunacy for Scotland. Paper Number: 3344, Volume/page: XXIII.457, CH Microfiche Number: 70.184-187:1-254.

SCL. 1870. Twelfth Annual Report of the General Board of Commissioners in Lunacy for Scotland. Paper Number: C.88, Volume/page: XXXIV.457, CH Microfiche Number: 76.346-349:1-284.

SCL. 1873. Fifteenth Annual Report of the General Board of Commissioners in Lunacy for Scotland. Paper Number: C.790, Volume/page: XXX.515,

CH Microfiche Number: 79.250-253:1-324.

SCL. 1876. Eighteenth Annual Report of the General Board of Commissioners in Lunacy for Scotland. Paper Number: C.1564, Volume/page: XLI.565, CH Microfiche Number: 83.304-306:1-208.

SCL. 1877. Nineteenth Annual Report of the General Board of Commissioners in Lunacy for Scotland. Paper Number: C.1785, Volume/page: XLI.773, CH Microfiche Number: 83.306-308:1-217.

SCL. 1878. Twentieth Annual Report of the general board of commissioners in lunacy for Scotland. Paper Number: C.2119, Volume/page: XXXIX.499, CH Microfiche Number: 84.293-295:1-196.

SCL. 1881. Twenty-third Annual Report of the General Board of Commissioners in Lunacy for Scotland. Paper Number: C.3023, Volume/page: XLVIII.569, CH Microfiche Number: 87.419-421: 1-202.

SCL. 1883. Twenty-fifth Annual Report of the General Board of Commissioners in Lunacy for Scotland. Paper Number: C.3779, Volume/page: XXX.611, CH Microfiche Number: 89.245-248:1-276.

SCL. 1884. Twenty-sixth Annual Report of the General Board of Commissioners in Lunacy for Scotland. 1884. Paper Number: C.4110, Volume/page: XL.559, CH Microfiche Number: 90.360-362: 1-239.

SCL. 1887. Twenty-ninth Annual Report of the General Board of Commissioners in Lunacy for Scotland. Paper Number: C.5093, Volume/page: XXXIX.399, CH Microfiche Number: 93.317-319:1-193.

SCL. 1891. Thirty-third Annual Report of the general board of commissioners in lunacy for Scotland. Paper Number: C.6441, Volume/page: XXXVI.341, CH Microfiche Number: 97.291-293:1-181.

SCL. 1892. Thirty-fourth Annual Report of the General Board of Commissioners in Lunacy for Scotland. Paper Number: C.6756, Volume/page: XL.549, CH Microfiche Number: 98.352-355:1-187.

SCL. 1900. Forty-second Annual Report of the General Board of Commissioners in Lunacy for Scotland. Paper Number: Cd.368, Volume/page: XXXVII.843, CH Microfiche Number: 106.330-333:1-251.

SCL. 1903. Forty-fifth Annual Report of the General Board of Commissioners in Lunacy for Scotland. Paper Number: Cd. 1539, Volume/page: XXVIII.1, CH Microfiche Number: 109.240:1-268.

SCL. 1905. Forty-seventh Annual Report of the General Board of Commissioners in Lunacy for Scotland. Paper Number: Cd. 2504, Volume/page: XXXVI.1, CH Microfiche Number: 111.327:1-276.

SCL. 1911. Fifty-third Annual Report of the General Board of Commissioners in Lunacy for Scotland. Paper Number: Cd. 5720, Volume/page: XXXV.207, CH Microfiche Number: 117.331: 1-268.

Primary sources Chapter Five

Laing, Ronald David. 1984. "Wisdom, Madness and Folly: The Making of a Psychiatrist 1927-1960." Papers of R.D. Laing, Special Collections, University of Glasgow. MS Laing A412.

Laing, Ronald David. 1980. "Oxford Companion to the Mind." Papers of R.D. Laing, Special Collections, University of Glasgow. MS Laing A575.

Laing, Ronald David. 1967a. "Seminar at the William Alanson White Institute, New York." Papers of R.D. Laing, Special Collections, University of Glasgow. MS Laing A262.

Laing, Ronald David. 1957/1981. "The Development of Ontological Security." Papers of R.D. Laing, Special Collections, University of Glasgow. MS Laing A586.

Laing, Ronald David. 1955. "The Rumpus Room." Papers of R.D. Laing, Special Collections, University of Glasgow. MS Laing A153.

References

Abrahamson, David. 2007. "RD Laing and long-stay patients: discrepant accounts of the refractory ward and 'rumpus room' at Gartnavel Royal Hospital." *History of Psychiatry* 18 (2):203-215.

Adams, Annmarie. 2007. "'That was then, this is now': Hospital architecture in the age(s) of revolution, 1970–2001." In *The Impact of Hospitals 300-2000*, edited by John Henderson, Peregrine Horden and Alessandro Pastore, 219-234. Oxford: Peter Lang.

Alexander, Christopher, Sara Ishikawa, and Murray Silverstein. 1977. *A Pattern Language: Towns, Buildings, Construction*. New York: Oxford University Press.

Algase, Donna L, Elizabeth RA Beattie, Cathy Antonakos, Cynthia A Beel-Bates, and Lan Yao. 2010. "Wandering and the physical environment." *American Journal of Alzheimer's Disease and Other Dementias* 25 (4):340-346.

Allen, John. 2003. *Lost Geographies of Power*. Malden, USA: Blackwell Publishing.

Åman, Anders. 1976. *Om den Offentliga Vården: Byggnader och Verksamheter vid Svenska Vårdinsitutioner under 1800-och 1900-talen. En Arkitekturhistorisk Undersökning*. [About public welfare ... An architectural investigation]. Stockholm: Liber Förlag: Arkitektur-museum.

Anderson, Ben. 2006. "Becoming and being hopeful: towards a theory of affect." *Environment and Planning D: Society and Space* 24 (5):733-752.

Anderson, Ben. 2009. "Affective atmospheres." *Emotion, Space and Society* 2 (2):77-81.

Anderson, Ben, and Paul Harrison. 2010a. "The promise of non-representational theories." In *Taking-Place: Non-Representational Theories and Geography*, edited by Ben Anderson and Paul Harrison, 2-34. Farnham: Ashgate.

Anderson, Ben, and Paul Harrison, eds. 2010b. *Taking-Place: Non-Representational Theories and Geography*. Farnham: Ashgate.

Anderson, Ben, and John Wylie. 2009. "On geography and materiality." *Environment and Planning A* 41 (2):318-335.

Anderson, Kay, and Susan J Smith. 2001. "Editorial: emotional geographies." *Transactions of the Institute of British Geographers* 26 (1):7-10.

Andersson, Jonas E. 2011. "*Architecture and Ageing: On the Interaction Between Frail Older People and the Built Environment.*" PhD diss., Dep. of Architecture and the Built Environment, KTH.

Andersson, Morgan. 2013. "*Användning och användbarhet i särskilda boendeformer för äldre.*" [Use and usability in assisted living facilities for older people] PhD diss., Department of Architecture, Chalmers University of Technology.

Andersson, Morgan, Nina Ryd, and Inga Malmqvist. 2014. "Exploring the function and use of common spaces in assisted living for older persons." *HERD: Health Environments Research & Design Journal* 7 (3):98-119.

Anderzhon, Jeffrey W, Ingrid L Fraley, and Mitch Green. 2007. *Design for Aging Post-Occupancy Evaluations: Lessons Learned from Senior Living Environments Featured in the AIA's Design for Aging Review*. Vol. 8. Hoboken NJ: John Wiley & Sons.

Andrews, Johnathan 1998. "R.D. Laing in Scotland: Facts and Fictions of the 'Rumpus Room' and Interpersonal Psychiatry." In *Cultures of Psychiatry and Mental Health Care in Postwar Britain and the Netherland*, edited by Marland Gijswijt-Hofstra and R Ponter, 121-150. Amsterdam: Rodopi.

Andrews, Johnathan, and Iain Smith, eds. 1993. *'Let There Be Light Again': A History of Gartnavel Royal Hospital from its beginnings to the present day*. Essays written to mark the 150th Anniversary in 1993 of Gartnavel Royal Hospital's existence on its present site.

Asdal, Kristin, Brita Brenna, and Ingunn Moser, eds. 2001. *Technosciense: The Politics of Interventions*. Oslo: Unipub.

Atkinson, Paul, and Amanda Coffey, eds. 2001. *Handbook of Ethnography*.

London: Sage.

Baker, Mona. 2006. *Translation and Conflict. A Narrative Account*. Oxon: Routledge.

Ballantyne, Andrew. 2004. "Misprisions of Stonehenge." In *Architecture as Experience: Radical Change in Spatial Practice* edited by Dana Arnold and Andrew Ballantyne, 11-35. London: Routledge.

Ballantyne, Andrew, and Chris L Smith. 2012. "Fluxions." In *Architecture in the Space of Flows*, edited by Andrew Ballantyne and Chris L Smith, 1-39. London: Routledge.

Barad, Karen. 2003. "Posthumanist performativity: Toward an understanding of how matter comes to matter." *Signs* 28 (3):801-831.

Barad, Karen. 2007. *Meeting the Universe Halfway: Quantum Physics and the Entanglement of Matter and Meaning*. Durham, NC: Duke University Press.

Barlas, David, Andrew E Sama, Mary F Ward, and Martin L Lesser. 2001. "Comparison of the auditory and visual privacy of emergency department treatment areas with curtains versus those with solid walls." *Annals of Emergency Medicine* 38 (2):135-139.

Barnes, Marian. 2012. *Care in Everyday Life: An Ethic of Care in Practice*. Bristol: Policy Press.

Barnes, Marian, Tula Brannelly, Lizzie Ward, and Nicki Ward. 2015. "Introduction: the critical significance of care." In *Ethics of Care: Critical Advances in International Perspective*, edited by Marian Barnes, Tula Brannelly, Lizzie Ward and Nicki Ward, 3-19. Bristol: Policy Press

Barrett, Peter, and Catherine A Stanley. 1999. *Better Construction Briefing*. Oxford: Blackwell.

Bauman, Zygmunt. 1991. *Modernity and Ambivalence*. Oxford: Polity Press.

BBR. 2015. *Regelsamling för Byggande*. BBR [Building regulations]. Karlskrona: The Swedish National Board of Housing, Building and Planning.

Beauchamp, Tom L, and James F Childress. 2001. *Principles of Biomedical Ethics*. Oxford: Oxford University Press.

Bennett, Jane. 2001. *The Enchantment of Modern Life: Attachments, Crossings, and Ethics*. Princeton, NJ: Princeton University Press.

Bennett, Jane. 2009. *Vibrant Matter: A Political Ecology of Things*. Durham: Duke University Press.

Berggren, Bengt, and Johan Cullberg. 1978. *Nacka Projektet - Bakgrund Praktik Erfarenhet. SPRI rapport 7 78*. [The Nacka project. Background, practice, experience]. Stockholm: SPRI Sjukvårdens och socialvårdens planerings- och rationaliseringsinstitut.

Berridge, David, Cherilyn Dance, Jennifer K Beecham, and Sarah Field. 2008. *Educating Difficult Adolescents. Effective Education for Children in Public Care or with Emotional and Behavioural Difficulties.* London: Jessica Kingsley Publishers.

Beveridge, Allan. 2011. *Portrait of the Psychiatrist as a Young Man: The Early Writing and Work of R.D. Laing, 1927-1960.* Oxford: Oxford University Press.

Beyes, Timon, and Chris Steyaert. 2011. "Spacing organization: non-representational theory and performing organizational space." *Organization* 19 (1):45-61.

BFS. 1993. *Nybyggnadsregler ändringar 1993:21* [New construction regulations, alterations]. Karlskrona: The Swedish National Board of Housing, Building and Planning.

Bissell, David. 2010. "Placing affective relations: Uncertain geographies of pain." In *Taking-Place: Non-Representational Theories and Geography*, edited by Ben Anderson and Paul Harrison, 79-97. Farnham: Ashgate.

Björgvinsson, Erling, and Gunnar Sandin. 2015. "Patients making place. A photography-based intervention about appropriation of hospital spaces." In *Art + Design + Architecture 6/2015, proceedings of the ARCH14 International Conference on Research on Health Care Architecture*, edited by Ira Verma and Laura Nenonen, 25-42. Helsinki: Aalto University publication series.

Blakstad, Siri H, Geir K Hansen, and Wibeke Knudsen. 2008. "Methods and tools for evaluation of usability in buildings." In *Usability of Workplaces, Phase 2*, edited by Keith Alexander. Rotterdam: CIB International Council for Research and Innovation in Building and Construction.

Blakstad, Siri Hunnes. 2001. "*A Strategic Approach to Adaptability in Office Buildings.*" PhD diss., Faculty of Architecture and Fine Art, NTNU.

Blyth, Alastair, and John Worthington. 2001. *Managing the Brief for Better Design.* London: Spon.

Bondi, Liz, and Joyce Davidson. 2011. "Lost in translation." *Transactions of the Institute of British Geographers* 36 (4):595-598.

Bordo, Susan, Binnie Klein, and Marilyn K Silverman. 1998. "Missing kitchens." In *Places Through the Body*, edited by Heidi J Nast and Steve Pile, 72-92. London: Routledge.

Brott, Simone. 2013a. *Architecture for a Free Subjectivity: Deleuze and Guattari at the Horizon of the Real*: Ashgate Publishing.

Brott, Simone. 2013b. "Toward a theory of the architectural subject." In *Deleuze and Architecture*, edited by Hélène Frichot and Stephen Loo, 151-167. Edinburgh: Edingburg University Press.

Böhme, Gernot. 1993. "Atmosphere as the fundamental concept of a new aesthetics." *Thesis Eleven* 36 (1):113-126.

Cache, Bernard. 1995. *Earth Moves*. London: The MIT Press.

Callon, Michel. 1986. "Some elements of a sociology of translation: domestication of the scallops and the fishermen of St Breuc Bay." In *Power, Action and Belief. A New Sociology of Knowledge*, edited by John Law, 196-233. London: Routledge & Kegan Paul.

Callon, Michel. 1996. "Le travail de la conception en architecture." *Situations. Les Cahiers de la Recherche Architecturale* (37):25-35.

Cameron, John. L, Ronald David Laing, and Andrew McGhie. 1955. "Patient and nurse: Effects of environmental changes in the care of chronic schizophrenics." *The Lancet:* 266 (6905):1384-1386

Carpman, Janet Reizenstein, Myron A Grant, and Deborah A Simmons. 1993. *Design that Cares: Planning Health Facilities for Patients and Visitors*. 2nd ed. Chicago: American Hospital Publishing.

Chantraine, Gilles. 2010. "French prisons of yesteryear and today: Two conflicting modernities-a socio-historical view." *Punishment & Society* 12 (1):27-46.

Clay, John. 1996. *R.D. Laing: A Divided Self*. London: Hodder & Stoughton.

Conradson, David. 2003. "Geographies of care: spaces, practices, experiences." *Social & Cultural Geography* 4 (4):451-454.

Conradson, David. 2005. "Landscape, care and the relational self: therapeutic encounters in rural England." *Health & Place* 11 (4):337-348.

Crafoord, Clarence. 1987. *Den Möjliga och Omöjliga Psykiatrin: Utveckling och Erfarenheter av Sektoriserad Psykiatri*. [The possible and impossible psychiatry: Development and experiences of decentralized psychiatry]. Stockholm: Natur och Kultur.

Cresswell, Tim. 2004. *Place: A Short Introduction*. Oxford: Blackwell Publishing.

Crouch, David. 2010. "Flirting with space: thinking landscape relationally." *Cultural Geographies* 17 (1):5-18.

Cuff, Dana. 2012. "Introduction: Architecture's double-bind." In *The SAGE Handbook of Architectural Theory*, edited by Greig Crysler, Stephen Cairns and Hilde Heynen, 385-393. London: Sage.

Cullberg, Johan. 2007. *Mitt Psykiatriska Liv: Memoarer*. [My psychiatric life: Memoirs]. Stockholm: Natur och Kultur.

Dawney, Leila. 2011. "The motor of being: a response to Steve Pile's 'Emotions and affect in recent human geography'." *Transactions of the Institute of British Geographers* 36 (4):599-602.

Degen, Monica, Gillian Rose, and Begum Basdas. 2010. "Bodies and everyday practices in designed urban environments." *Science Studies* 23 (2):60-76.

Delamont, Sara. 2004. "Ethnography and participant observation." In *Qualitative Research Practice*, edited by Clive Seale, Giampietro Gobo, Jaber F Gubrium and David Silverman, 205-217. London: Sage.

DeLanda, Manuel. 2006. *A New Philosophy of Society. Assemblage Theory and Social Complexity*. London: Bloomsbury.

Deleuze, Gilles. 1988. *Foucault*. Minneapolis: University of Minnesota Press.

Deleuze, Gilles, and Felix Guattari. 1986. *Nomadology: The War Machine* Translated by Brian Massumi. New York: Semiotext(e) Original edition, Traité de nomadologie.

Deleuze, Gilles, and Félix Guattari. 1994. *What is Philosophy?* New York: Columbia University Press.

Deleuze, Gilles, and Félix Guattari. 2004. *A Thousand Plateaus: Capitalism and Schizophrenia*. London: Continuum.

Dewsbury, John David. 2000. "Performativity and the event: enacting a philosophy of difference." *Environment and Planning D: Society and Space* 18:473-496.

Dewsbury, John David, Paul Harrison, Mitch Rose, and John Wylie. 2002. "Enacting geographies." *Geoforum* 33 (4):437-440.

Doel, Marcus A. 2000. "Un-glunking geography. Spatial science after Dr. Seuss and Gilles Deleuze." In *Thinking space*, edited by Mike Crang and Nigel Thrift, 117-135. London: Routledge.

Doel, Marcus A. 2010. "Representation and difference." In *Taking-Place: Non-Representational Theories and Geography*, edited by Ben Anderson and Paul Harrison, 117-130. Farnham: Ashgate.

Doucet, Isabelle, and Kenny Cupers. 2009. "Agency and architecture: Rethinking criticality in theory and practice." *Footprint* 8 (Spring):1-6.

Douglas, Calbert H, and Mary R Douglas. 2004. "Patient-friendly hospital environments: exploring the patients' perspective." *Health Expectations* 7 (1):61-73.

Dovey, Kim. 2008. *Framing Places: Mediating Power in Built Form*. 2nd ed. London: Routledge.

Dovey, Kim. 2013. "Assembling architecture." In *Deleuze and Architecture*, edited by Hélène Frichot and Stephen Loo. Edinburgh: Edinburgh University Press.

Eliasson-Lappalainen, Rosmarie. 1979. *Den Nya Psykiatrin i Korseld: En Rapport från Skå om Nacka-projektet, Psykoterapi och Ideologi*. [Crossfiring the new psychiatry: a report from Skå on the Nacka Project, psycho-therapy and ideology]. Stockholm: Prisma.

Evans, Robin. 1978. "Figures, doors and passages." *Architectural Design* 48 (4):267-278.

Evans, Simon, and Sarah Vallelly. 2007. *Best Practice in Promoting Social Well-being in Extra Care Housing: A Literature Review*. York: Joseph Rowntree Foundation.

Fairless, W. D. 1861. *Suggestions Concerning the Construction of Asylums for the Insane*. Edinburgh: Royal College of Physicians.

Fairweather, Leslie, and Sean McConville, eds. 2000. *Prison Architecture: Policy, Design, and Experience*. Oxford: Architectural Press.

Fenwick, Tara, and Paolo Landri. 2012. "Materialities, textures and pedagogies: socio-material assemblages in education." *Pedagogy, Culture & Society* 20 (1):1-7.

Foucault, Michel. 1961. *Histoire de la Folie à l'Age Classique*. Paris: Plon.

Foucault, Michel. 1965. *Madness and Civilization: A History of Insanity in the Age of Reason* Edited by (abridged English edition). New York: Pantheon.

Foucault, Michel. 1970. *The Order of Things: an Archaeology of the Human Sciences*. London: Pantheon Books.

Foucault, Michel. 1977. *Discipline and Punish: The Birth of the Prison*. New York: Vintage.

Foucault, Michel. 1981. *The History of Sexuality, Vol.1: An Introduction*. Harmondsworth: Penguin.

Foucault, Michel. 1982. "The subject and power." *Critical inquiry* 8 (4):777-795.

Foucault, Michel. 2006. *Psychiatric Power: Lectures at the Collège de France, 1973-1974*. Translated by Graham Burchell. Basingstoke: Palgrave Macmillan.

Frankowski, Ann Christine, Erin G Roth, J Kevin Eckert, and Brandy Harris-Wallace. 2011. "The dining room as locus of ritual in assisted living." *Generations* 35 (3):41.

Freeman, Thomas, John L Cameron, and Andrew McGhie. 1958. *Chronic Schizophrenia*. New York: International Universities Press.

Frichot, Helene. 2005. "Stealing into Deleuze's baroque house." In *Deleuze and Space*, edited by Ian Buchanan and Gregg Lambert, 61-79. Edinburgh: Edinburgh University Press.

Galison, Peter. 1997. *Image and Logic: A Material Culture of Microphysics*. Chicago: University of Chicago Press.

Garfinkel, Harold. 1967. *Studies in Ethnomethodology*. Englewood Cliffs: Prentice Hall.

Gleeson, Brendan, and Robin Kearns. 2001. "Remoralising landscapes of care." *Environment and Planning D: Society and Space* 19 (1):61-80.

Godfrey, Walter Hindes. 1955. *The English Almshouse: With Some Account of its Predecessor, the Medieval Hospital*. London: Faber & Faber.

Goffman, Erving. 1961. *Asylums: Essays on the Social Situation of Mental Patients and Other Inmates*. New York: Penguin Books.

Goffman, Erving. 1986. *Frame Analysis: An Essay on the Organization of Experience*. Boston: Northeastern University Press. Original edition, 1974.

Graham, Stephen, and Nigel Thrift. 2007. "Out of order: Understanding repair and maintenance." *Theory, Culture & Society* 24 (3):1-25.

Granath, Jan-Åke. 1991. "Architecture, Technology and Human Factors: Design in a Socio-Technical Context."PhD diss., Dep. of Architecture, Chalmers University of Technology.

Grosz, Elisabeth. 2001. *Architecture From the Outside. Essays on Virtual and Real Space*. Cambridge, Mass.: MIT Press.

Harvey, David. 2006. *Spaces of Global Capitalism*. London: Verso.

Hauge, Solveig, and Kirsten Heggen. 2008. "The nursing home as a home: a field study of residents' daily life in the common living rooms." *Journal of Clinical Nursing* 17 (4):460-467.

Hetherington, Kevin. 1997. *The Badlands of Modernity: Heterotopia and Social Ordering*. London: Routledge.

Hillier, Jean, and Gareth Abrahams. 2013. "Deleuze and Guattari. Jean Hillier in conversation with Gareth Abrahams." In: AESOP. www.aesop-planning.eu (accessed 2016-01-06).

Houdart, Sophie. 2008. "Copying, cutting and pasting social spheres." *Science Studies: An Interdisciplinary Journal of Science and Technology* 21 (1):47-63.

Houdart, Sophie, and Chihiro Minato. 2009. *Kuma Kengo: An Unconventional Monograph*. Paris: Editions Donner Lieu.

Hurdley, Rachel. 2010. "The power of corridors: connecting doors, mobilising materials, plotting openness." *The Sociological Review* 58 (1):45-64.

Högström, Ebba. 2012. "*Kalejdoskopiska Rum: Diskurs, Materialitet och Praktik i den Decentraliserade Psykiatriska Vården*." [Kaleidoscopic spaces. Discourse, materiality and practice in decentralised mental healthcare] PhD diss., Dep. of Architecture and the Built Environment, Royal Institute of Technology.

ISO. 1998. *Ergonomic Requirements for Office Work with Visual Display*

Terminals (VDTs). Part 11: ISO 9241-11:1998. Guidance on Usability. Genève: International Organization of Standardization.

Jackson, Alecia Youngblood. 2013. "Posthumanist data analysis of mangling practices." *International Journal of Qualitative Studies in Education* 26 (6):741-748.

Jacobs, Jane M. 2006. "A geography of big things." *Cultural Geographies* 13 (1):1-27.

Jacobs, Jane M, Stephen Cairns, and Ignaz Strebel. 2007. "'A tall storey ... but, a fact just the dame': The red road high-rise as a black box." *Urban Studies* 44 (3):609-629.

Jacobs, Jane M, and Peter Merriman. 2011. "Practising architectures." *Social & Cultural Geography* 12 (3):211-222.

Jeffrey, Alex, Colin McFarlane, and Alex Vasudevan. 2012. "Rethinking enclosure: Space, subjectivity and the commons." *Antipode* 44 (4):1247-1267.

Jersild, Per Christian. 2015. *Den Stökiga Psykiatrin: Minnen, Samtal, tankar.* [The messy psychiatry: memories, dialogues, thoughts]. Lidingö: Fri tanke.

Jones, Geoff, Christine McLean, and Paolo Quattrone. 2004. "Spacing and timing." *Organization* 11 (6):723-741.

Jönsson, Catharina. 1991. *Vers une Cuisine Améliorée: une Etude sur Les Cuisines et les Foyers Dans le Cadre du Project UNSO Foyers Améliorés au Burkina Faso.* Lund: Lund Centre for Habitat Studies.

King, Steven. 2013. "Introduction: Hertfordshire in context." In *Social Welfare in Hertfordshire from 1600: A Caring County?*, edited by Steven King and Gillian Gear, 1-13. Hertfordshire, UK: University of Hertfordshire Press.

Korosec-Serfaty, Perla. 1973. "The Case of Newly Constructed Zones: Freedom, Constraint and the Appropriation of Spaces." *Architectural Psychology, proceedings of the Lund Conference*, edited by Richard Küller, 392-393. Lund: Studentlitteratur.

Kraftl, Peter. 2010. "Geographies of architecture: the multiple lives of buildings." *Geography Compass* 4 (5):402-415.

Kraftl, Peter, and Peter Adey. 2008. "Architecture/Affect/Inhabitation: Geographies of Being-In Buildings." *Annals of the Association of American Geographers* 98 (1):213-231.

Kuhn, Thomas. 1962. *The Structure of Scientific Revolutions.* Chicago: University of Chicago Press.

Laing, Ronald David. 1985. *Wisdom, Madness and Folly: the Making of a Psychiatrist 1927-1957.* London: Macmillan.

Laing, Ronald David. (1960) 1969. *The Divided Self: a Study of Sanity and*

Madness. London: Tavistock. Reprint, London: Penguin books. Citations refer to the Penguin edition.

Laing, Ronald David. (1969) 1972. *Self and Others*. 2nd ed. London: Tavistock. Reprint, London: Penguin Books. Citations refer to the Penguin edition.

Laing, Ronald David, and Aaron Esterson. (1964) 1970. *Sanity, Family and Madness*. 2nd ed. Vol. 1. Families of Schizophrenics. London: Tavistock. Reprint, London: Penguin Books. Citations refer to the Penguin edition.

Landrum, Timothy J, Melody Tankersley, and James M Kauffman. 2003. "What is special about special education for students with emotional or behavioral disorders?" *The Journal of Special Education* 37 (3):148-156.

Lash, Scott, Antoine Picon, Kenny Cupers, Isabelle Doucet, and Margaret Crawford. 2009. "Agency and architecture: how to be critical." *Footprint* 8 (Spring):7-19.

Latham, Alan, and Derek P McCormack. 2004. "Moving cities: rethinking the materialities of urban geographies." *Progress in Human Geography* 28 (6):701-724.

Latour, Bruno. 1984. "The powers of association." *The Sociological Review* 32 (S1):264-280.

Latour, Bruno. 2000. "When things strike back: a possible contribution of 'science studies' to the social sciences." *The British Journal of Sociology* 51 (1):107-123.

Latour, Bruno. 2005. *Reassembling the Social: An Introduction to Actor-Network-Theory*. Oxford: University Press.

Latour, Bruno, and Albena Yaneva. 2008. "Give me a gun and I will make all buildings move: An ANT's view of architecture " In *Explorations in Architecture: Teaching, Design, Research*, edited by Geiser; Reto, 80-89. Basel: Birkhäuser.

Law, John. 1994. *Organizing Modernity*. Oxford: Blackwell.

Law, John. 1999. "After ANT: complexity, naming and topology." *The Sociological Review* 47 (S1):1-14.

Law, John. 2004. *After Method: Mess in Social Science Research*. London: Routledge.

Laws, Jennifer. 2012. "'Working Through': An Inquiry into Work and Madness. "Unpublished PhD diss., School of Geography, Durham University, UK.

Lawson, Victoria. 2007. "Geographies of care and responsibility." *Annals of the Association of American Geographers* 97 (1):1-11.

Lees, Loretta. 2001. "Towards a critical geography of architecture: the case of an ersatz Colosseum." *Ecumene* 8 (1):51-86.

Lefebvre, Henri. 1991. *The Production of Space*. Oxford: Basil Blackwell.

Linwood, Anne. 2003. *Storthes Hall Remembered*. Huddersfield, UK: The University of Huddersfield.

Llewellyn, Mark. 2004. "'Urban village' or 'white house': envisioned spaces, experienced places, and everyday life at Kensal House, London in the 1930s." *Environment and Planning D: Society and Space* 22 (2):229-249.

Lorimer, Hayden. 2007. "Cultural geography: worldly shapes, differently arranged." *Progress in Human Geography* 31 (1):89-100.

Lorimer, Hayden. 2008. "Cultural geography: non-representational conditions and concerns." *Progress in Human Geography* 32 (4):551-559.

Loukissas, Yanni Alexander. 2012. *Co-designers: Cultures of Computer Simulation in Architecture*. London: Routledge.

Lynch, Michael. 1985. "Discipline and the material form of images: An analysis of scientific visibility." *Social Studies of Science* 15 (1):37-66.

Lynch, Michael. 1993. *Scientific Practice and Ordinary Action: Ethnomethodology and Social Studies of Science*. Cambridge: Cambridge University Press.

Lynch, Michael, and Steve Woolgar. 1990. *Representation in Scientific Practice*. Cambridge, MA: MIT Press.

Lynch, Michel, and Samuel Y Edgerton. 1988. "Aesthetics and digital image processing: Representational craft in contemporary astronomy." In *Picturing Power: Visual Depiction and Social Relations*, edited by Gordon Fyte and John Law, 184-220. London: Routledge.

Malabou, Catherine. 2010. *Plasticity at the Dusk of Writing: Dialectic, Destruction, Deconstruction*. New York: Columbia University Press.

Malabou, Catherine. 2012. *Ontology of the Accident, an Essay on Destructive Plasticity.* Cambridge/Malden: Polity Press,.

Malabou, Catherine. 2015. "After the flesh." In *Plastic Bodies: Rebuilding Sensation After Phenomenology*, edited by Tom Sparrow, 13-20. London: Open Humanities Press.

Marcus, George E, and Erkan Saka. 2006. "Assemblage." *Theory, Culture & Society* 23 (2-3):101-106.

Markus, Thomas A. 1993. *Buildings & Power: Freedom and Control in the Origin of Modern Building Types*. London: Psychology Press.

Markus, Thomas A, and Deborah Cameron. 2002. *The Words Between the Spaces: Buildings and Language*. London: Routledge.

Martin, Biddy, and Chandra Talpade Mohanty. 1986. "Feminist politics: What's home got to do with it?" In *Feminist Studies/Cultural Studies*, edited by Teresa de Lauretis, 293-310.

Massey, Doreen. 2005. *For Space*. London: Sage.

Massumi, Brian. 2002. *Parables for the Virtual*. Durham: Duke University Press.

McCormack, Brendan, and Tanya McCance. 2011. *Person-Centred Nursing: Theory and Practice*. Chichester, West Sussex: Wiley-Blackwell.

McCormack, Derek P. 2003. "An event of geographical ethics in spaces of affect." *Transactions of the Institute of British Geographers* 28 (4):488-507.

McCormack, Derek P. 2005. "Diagramming practice and performance." *Environment and Planning D: Society and Space* 23 (1):119-147.

McGeachan, Cheryl. 2013. "Needles, picks and an intern named Laing: exploring the psychiatric spaces of Army life." *Journal of Historical Geography* 40:67-78.

McGeachan, Cheryl. 2014. "'Worlding' psychoanalytic insights: unpicking R.D. Laing's geographies." In *Psychoanalytic Geographies*, edited by Paul Kingsbury and Steve Pile, 89-102. Farnham: Ashgate.

Merleau-Ponty, Maurice. 1962. *Phenomenology of Perception*. Translated by Colin Smith. London: Routledge. Original edition, Phénoménologie de la perception Paris, Gallimard, 1945.

Merrell, Floyd. 1996. "Vagueness, generality and undeciding otherness." In *Peirce's Doctrine of Signs: Theory, Applications, and Connections*, edited by Vincent M Colapietro and Thomas M Olshewsky, 35-43. Berlin/New York: Walter de Gruyter.

Miller, Gavin. 2004. *R.D. Laing*. Edinburgh: Edinburgh University Press.

Miller, Vincent. 2006. "The unmappable vagueness and spatial experience." *Space and Culture* 9 (4):453-467.

Milligan, Christine, and Janine Wiles. 2010. "Landscapes of care." *Progress in Human Geography* 34 (6):736-754.

Mol, Annemarie. 1999. "Ontological politics. A word and some questions." *The Sociological Review* 47 (S1):74-89.

Mol, Annemarie. 2010. "Care and its values. Good food in the nursing home." In *Care in Practice. On Tinkering in Clinics, Homes and Farms*, edited by Annemarie Mol, Ingunn Moser and Jeanette Pols, 215-234. Bielefeld: Transcript.

Mol, Annemarie, and John Law. 1994. "Regions, networks and fluids: anaemia and social topology." *Social Studies of Science* 24 (4):641-671.

Mol, Annemarie, Ingunn Moser, and Jeanette Pols, eds. 2010. *Care in Practice. On Tinkering in Clinics, Homes and Farms*. Bielefeld: Transcript.

Moore, Keith Diaz. 1999. "Dissonance in the dining room: A study of social interaction in a special care unit." *Quality Health Research* 9 (133-155).

Morrison, Hazel. 2014. "Unearthing the Clinical Encounter: Gartnavel Mental Hospital 1921 - 1932. Exploring the intersection of scientific and social discourses which negotiated the boundaries of psychiatric diagnoses."Unpublished PhD diss., Human Geography?, University of Glasgow.

Moser, Ingunn. 2005. "On becoming disabled and articulating alternatives: The multiple modes of ordering disability and their interferences." *Cultural Studies* 19 (6):667-700.

Moser, Ingunn. 2010a. "Diagnosing and acting upon dementia: Marte Meo." In *Ethnographies of Diagnostic Work*, edited by D Goodwin, J Mesman and M Buscher, 193-208. London: Palgrave University Press.

Moser, Ingunn. 2010b. "Perhaps tears should not be counted but wiped away. On quality and improvement in dementia care." In *Care in Practice. On Tinkering in Clinics, Homes and Farms*, edited by Annemarie Mol, Ingunn Moser and Jeanette Pols, 277-298. Bielefeld: Transcript.

Moser, Ingunn. 2011. "Dementia and the limits to life: anthropological sensibilities, STS interferences, and possibilities for action in care." *Science, Technology & Human Values* 36 (5):704-722.

Moser, Ingunn. 2016. "Sociotechnical practices and difference: On the interferences between disability, gender, and class." In *Rethinking DisAbility: World Perspectives in Culture and Society*, edited by Patrick Devlieger, Beatriz Miranda-Galarza, Steven E Brown and Megan Strickfaden, 405-426. Antwerp: Garant.

Moser, Ingunn. 2017. "Disability and the promises of technology: Technology, subjectivity and embodiment within an order of the normal." In *Disability, Space, Architecture. A Reader*, edited by J Boys. London: Routledge.

Moser, Ingunn, and John Law. 2007. "Good Passages. Bad Passages." In *Technoscience. The Politics of Interventions*, edited by Kristin Asdal, Brita Brenna and Ingunn Moser, 157-178. Oslo: Unipub.

Mullan, Bob. 1997. *R.D. Laing: Creative Destroyer.* London: Cassell.

Munro, Moira, and Ruth Madigan. 1999. "Negotiating space in the family home." In *At Home: An Anthropology of Domestic Space*, edited by Irene Cieraad, 107-117. Syracuse: Syracuse University Press.

Murdoch, Jonathan. 1998. "The spaces of actor-network theory." *Geoforum* 29 (4):357-374.

Nanda, Upali, Sarajane L Eisen, and Veerabhadran Baladandayuthapani. 2008. "Undertaking an art survey to compare patient versus student art preferences." *Environment and Behavior* 40 (2):269-301.

Nord, Catharina. 2011a. "Architectural space as a moulding factor of care practices and resident privacy in assisted living." *Ageing & Society* 31 (6):934-952.

Nord, Catharina. 2011b. "Individual care and personal space in assisted living in Sweden." *Health & Place* 17 (1):50-56.

Nord, Catharina. 2013a. "A day to be lived. Elderly peoples' possessions for everyday life in assisted living." *Journal of Aging Studies* 27 (2):135-142.

Nord, Catharina. 2013b. "Design according to the law: juridical dimensions of architecture for assisted living in Sweden." *Journal of Housing and the Built Environment* 28 (1):147-155.

Nord, Catharina. 2015. "Architectural space in respite and intermediate care–an Actor- Network Theory analysis " *Journal of Housing for the Elderly* 29 (1-2).

Ohlsson, Anna. 2008. "*Myt och Manipulation: Radikal Psykiatrikritik i Svensk Offentlig Idédebatt 1968-1973.*" [Myth and manipulation: Radical critic of phsychiatry in Swedish public debate 1968-1973] PhD diss., Dep. of Literature and the History of Ideas, Stockholm University.

Parr, Hester. 2008. *Mental Health and Social Space: Towards Inclusionary Geographies*. Oxford: Blackwell Publishing.

Peirce, Charles. 1902. Vague. In *Dictionary of Philosophy and Psychology*, edited by J.M. Baldwin. New York: MacMillan.

Philo, Chris. 2001. "Accumulating populations: bodies, institutions and space." *International Journal of Population Geography* 7 (6):473-490.

Philo, Chris. 2004. *A Geographical History of Institutional Provision for the Insane from Medieval Times to the 1860s in England and Wales: 'The Space Reserved for Insanity'*. Lewiston and Queenston, USA and Lampeter, UK: Edwin Mellen Press.

Philo, Chris. 2007. "Michel Foucault, Psychiatric Power: Lectures at the Collège de France 1973-1974." *Foucault Studies* 4:149-163.

Philo, Chris. 2012. "A 'new Foucault'with lively implications–or 'the crawfish advances sideways'." *Transactions of the Institute of British Geographers* 37 (4):496-514.

Philo, Chris. 2013. "'A great space of murmurings': Madness, romance and geography." *Progress in Human Geography* 37 (2):167-194.

Philo, Chris, and John Pickstone. 2009. "Unpromising configurations: towards local historical geographies of psychiatry." *Health & Place* 15 (3):649-656.

Pickering, Andrew, ed. 1992. *Science as Practice and Culture*. Chicago: University of Chicago Press.

Pickering, Andrew. 1993. "The mangle of practice: Agency and emergence in the sociology of science." *American Journal of Sociology* 99 (3):559-589.

Pile, Steve. 2010. "Emotions and affect in recent human geography." *Transactions of the Institute of British Geographers* 35 (1):5-20.

Pols, Jeannette. 2011. "Breathtaking practicalities: a politics of embodied patient positions." *Scandinavian Journal of Disability Research* 13 (3):189-206.

Pols, Jeannette. 2016. "Analyzing social spaces: Relational citizenship for patients leaving mental health care institutions." *Medical Anthropology* 35 (2):177.

Porter, Roy. 2002. *Madness: A Brief History.* Oxford: Oxford University Press.

Pryor, Eric. 1993. *Claybury: A Century of Caring.* Lavenham, Suffolk, UK: The Mental Health Care Group, Forest Healthcare Trust and The Lavenham Press Ltd.

Putnam, Tim. 1999. "'Postmodern' home life." In *At Home: An Anthropology of Domestic Space*, edited by Irene Cieraad, 144-152. Syracuse: Syracuse University Press.

Rancière, Jacques. 2005. "From politics to aesthetics?" *Paragraph* 28 (1):13-25.

Rasila, Heidi, Peggie Rothe, and Heidi Kerosuo. 2010. "Dimensions of usability assessment in built environments." *Journal of Facilities Management* 8 (2):143-153.

Regnier, Victor. 2002. *Design for Assisted Living. Guidelines for Housing the Physically and Mentally Frail.* New York: John Wiley and Sons.

Riggins, Stephen Harold. 1994. "Fieldwork in the living room: An autoethnographic essay." In *The Socialness of Things: Essays on the Socio-Semiotics of Objects*, edited by Stephen Harold Riggins, 101-147. Berlin: Mouton de Gruyter.

Rose, Gillian. 1993. *Feminism & Geography: The Limits of Geographical Knowledge.* Cambridge: Polity Press.

Ryd, Nina, and Sven Fristedt. 2007. "Transforming strategic briefing into project briefs: A case study about client and contractor collaboration." *Facilities* 25 (5/6):185-202.

Saarikangas, Kirsi. 2006. "Displays of the everyday. Relations between gender and the visibility of domestic work in the modern Finnish kitchen from the 1930s to the 1950s." *Gender, Place & Culture* 13 (2):161-172.

Sacks, Harvey. 1992. *Lectures on Conversation.* Vol. 1 and ll. Oxford: Blackwell.

Schillmeier, Michael, and Miquel Domenech, eds. 2010. *New Technologies and Emerging Spaces of Care*. Farnham: Ashgate.

Sandin, Gunnar. 2003. "Modalities of Place: On Polarisation and Exclusion in Concepts of Place and in Site-specific Art." PhD diss., Department of Architecture and Built Environment, Lund University.

Sandin, Gunnar. 2015. "Modes of transgression in institutional critique." In *Transgression: Towards an Expanded Field of Architecture*, edited by Louis Rice and David Littlefield, 217-229. London: Routledge.

Sandin, Gunnar, and Lars-Henrik Ståhl. 2011. "Aesthetic replacement strategies in hospitals." Paper presented at *Ambience 11: Where art, technology and design meet*, University of Borås, November 2011.

Schwarz, Benyamin. 1997. "Nursing home design: A misguided architectural model." *Journal of Architectural and Planning Research* 14 (4):343-359.

Schwarz, Benyamin, and Ruth Brent, eds. 1999. *Aging, Autonomy and Architecture: Advances in Assisted Living*. Baltimore: John Hopkins University Press.

Sedgwick, Eve Kosofsky. 2003. *Touching Feeling: Affect, Pedagogy, Performativity*. Durham: Duke University Press.

Severinsson, Susanne. 2010. "*Unga i Normalitetens Gränsland: Undervisning och Behandling i Särskilda Undervisningsgrupper och Hem för Vård eller Boende.*" [Adolescent in the borderland of normality: Education and treatment in special education classes and foster institutions] PhD diss., Dep. of Social and Welfare Studies, Linköping University.

Severinsson, Susanne. 2015. "Documentation for students in residential care: network of relations of human and non-human actants." *International Journal of Inclusive Education*:1-13.

Severinsson, Susanne, and Catharina Nord. 2015. "Emergent subjectivity in caring institutions for teenagers." *Pastoral Care in Education* 33 (3):137-146.

Severinsson, Susanne, Catharina Nord, and Eva Reimers. 2015. "Ambiguous spaces for troubled youth: home, therapeutic institution or school?" *Pedagogy, Culture & Society* 23 (2):245-264.

Sharp, Joanne. 2009. "Geography and gender: what belongs to feminist geography? Emotion, power and change." *Progress in Human Geography* 33 (1):74.

Sharp, Joanne P, Paul Routledge, Chris Philo, and Ronan Paddison, eds. 2000. *Entanglements of Power. Geographies of Domination/ Resistance*. London: Routledge.

Sibbald, John. 1897. *On the Plans of Modern Asylums for the Insane Poor*. Edinburgh: James Turner & Co.

Simonsen, Kirsten. 2005. "Bodies, sensations, space and time: The contribution from Henri Lefebvre." *Geografiska Annaler: Series B, Human Geography* 87 (1):1-14.

Sloane, David Charles. 1994. "Scientific paragon to hospital mall: the evolving design of the hospital, 1885–1994." *Journal of Architectural Education* 48 (2):82-98.

Smyth, John, Peter McInerney, and Tim Fish. 2013. "Blurring the boundaries: From relational learning towards a critical pedagogy of engagement for disengaged disadvantaged young people." *Pedagogy, Culture & Society* 21 (2):299-320.

Sommer, Robert. 1969. *Personal Space. The Behavioral Basis of Design.* Bristol: Bosko Books.

Sorensen, Roy. 2001. *Vagueness and Contradiction.* Oxford: Clarendon Press.

Sorensen, Roy. 2012. "Vagueness". *The Stanford Encyclopedia of Philosophy.* Accessed 20151010.

Spandler, Helen. 2009. "Spaces of psychiatric contention: A case study of a therapeutic community." *Health & Place* 15 (3):672-678.

Spierenburg, Pieter. 1984. "Introduction." In *The Emergence of Carceral Institutions: Prisons, Galleys and Lunatic Asylums, 1550-1900*, edited by Pieter Spierenburg, 2-8. Rotterdam: Erasmus University (Centrum voor Maatschappij Geschiedenis).

SPRI. 1981. *Nackaprojektet - Öppenvårdslokaler för Psykiatri: Delrapport 1: Probleminventering, Kravanalys. SPRI Rapport 54.* [The Nacka project-Spaces for psychiatric outpatient care. Part-time report 1: problem inventory, requirement analysis. SPRI report 54]. Stockholm: SPRI Sjukvårdens och socialvårdens planerings- och rationaliseringsinstitut.

SPRI. 1983. *Nackaprojektet - Öppenvårdslokaler för Psykiatri: Delrapport 2: Diskussionsunderlag vid Planering, SPRI Rapport 114.* [The Nacka project-Spaces for psychiatric outpatient care. Part-time report 2. SPRI report 114]. Stockholm: SPRI Sjukvårdens och socialvårdens planerings- och rationaliseringsinstitut.

SPRI. 1985. *Lokaler för Psykiatri. SPRI Rapport 101.* [Facilites for psychiatry. SPRI report 101]. Stockholm: SPRI Sjukvårdens och socialvårdens planerings- och rationaliseringsinstitut.

Stander, Marcus, Aristotelis Hadjakos, Niklas Lochschmidt, Christian Klos, Bastian Renner, and Max Muhlhauser. 2012. "A Smart Kitchen Infrastructure." *2013 IEEE International Symposium on Multimedia*, 96-99.

Strebel, Ignaz. 2011. "The living building: Towards a geography of maintenance work." *Social & Cultural Geography* 12 (03):243-262.

Street, Alice. 2012. "Affective Infrastructure: Hospital Landscapes of Hope and Failure." *Space and Culture* 15 (1):44-56.

Sullivan, Harry Stack 1955. *The Interpersonal Theory of Psychiatry*. London: Tavistock Publications.

Szecsödy, Imre, Maria Hansson, Marie Hessle, and Ulf Nordahl. 1980. "Architectural boundaries and their impact on social organizations." In *The Individual and the Group: Boundaries and Interrelations*, edited by Malcolmand Pines and Lise Rafaelsen, 307-320. Springer.

Thien, Deborah. 2005. "After or beyond feeling? A consideration of affect and emotion in geography." *Area* 37 (4):450-454.

Thrift, Nigel. 2004. "Intensities of feeling: towards a spatial politics of affect." *Geografiska Annaler: Series B, Human Geography* 86 (1):57-78.

Thrift, Nigel. 2006. "Space." *Theory, Culture & Society* 23 (2-3):139-146.

Thrift, Nigel. 2008. *Non-Representational Theory: Space, Politics, Affect*. London: Routledge.

Till, Jeremy. 2009. *Architecture Depends*. Cambridge, Mass: MIT press.

Toila-Kelly, Divya P. 2006. "Affect-an ethnocentric encounter? Exploring the universalist imperative of emotional/affectual geographies." *Area* 38 (2):213-217.

Tomes, Nancy. 1994. *The Art of Asylum Keeping: Thomas Story Kirkbride and the Origins of American Psychiatry*. Philadelphia: University of Pennsylvania Press.

Topp, Leslie Elizabeth, James E Moran, and Jonathan Andrews, eds. 2007. *Madness, Architecture and the Built Environment: Psychiatric Spaces in Historical Context*. New York, London: Routledge.

Trefry, John H, and Laurel B Watson. 2013. "The silenced voices of architectural discourse: promoting inclusion through qualitative research." *Enquiry: A Journal for Architectural Research* 10 (1):10.

Tronto, Joan C. 1993. *Moral Boundaries: A Political Argument for an Ethic of Care*. London: Routledge.

Tschumi, Bernhard. 1996. *Architecture and Disjunction*. Cambridge, Mass: MIT Press.

Tuan, Yi-Fu. 1991. "A view of geography." *Geographical Review* 81 (1):99-107.

Ulrich, Roger. 2001. "Effects of healthcare environmental design on medical outcomes." In *Design and Health: Proceedings of the Second International Conference on Health and Design,* 49-59. Stockholm: Svensk Byggtjänst.

Ulrich, Roger. 2006. "Essay: evidence-based health-care architecture." *The*

Lancet 368:S38-S39.

Ulrich, Roger S, Craig Zimring, Xiaobo Quan, Anjali Joseph, and Ruchi Choudhary. 2004. "The role of the physical environment in the hospital of the 21st Century: An once-in-a-lifetime opportunity." In *Report to The Center for Health Design for the Designing the 21st Century Hospital Project.* Center of Health Design.

Unwin, F.T. 1976. *Dew on My Feet.* Ilfracombe, UK: Arthur H. Stockwell Ltd.

Upitis, Rena. 2004. "School architecture and complexity." *Complicity: An International Journal of Complexity and Education* 1 (1):19-38.

Wagenaar, Coor, ed. 2006. *The Architecture of Hospitals.* Rotterdam: Nai Publishers.

Walch, Jeffrey M, Bruce S Rabin, Richard Day, Jessica N Williams, Krissy Choi, and James D Kang. 2005. "The effect of sunlight on postoperative analgesic medication use: a prospective study of patients undergoing spinal surgery." *Psychosomatic Medicine* 67 (1):156-163.

Vale, Lawrence. 2014. *Architecture, Power and National Identity.* 2nd ed. London: Routledge.

Walker, Anthony. 2015. *Project Management in Construction.* 6th ed. Oxford: Wiley-Blackwell.

Warell, Anders. 2001. "*Design Syntactics: A Functional Approach to Visual Product form Theory, Models, and Methods.*" PhD diss., Dep. of Architecture, Chalmers University of Technology.

Wetherell, Margaret. 2012. *Affect and Emotion: A New Social Science Understanding.* London: Sage.

Wigley, Mark. 1993. *The Architecture of Deconstruction: Derrida's Haunt.* Cambridge, Mass.: MIT Press

Willmann, Marc. 2007. "The forgotten schools. Current status of special schools for pupils with social, emotional and behavioural difficulties in Germany: A complete national survey." *Emotional and Behavioural Difficulties* 12 (4):299-318.

Winnicott, Donald W. 2003. *Lek och Verklighet* Translated by Ingeborg Löfgren. 3rd ed. Stockholm: Natur och Kultur. Original edition, Playing and reality.

Wolch, Jennifer, and Chris Philo. 2000. "From distributions of deviance to definitions of difference: past and future mental health geographies." *Health & Place* 6 (3):137-157.

Wolpert, Julian. 1976. "Opening closed spaces." *Annals of the Association of American Geographers* 66 (1):1-13.

Wright, Anne-Marie. 2009. "Every child matters: Discourses of challenging behaviour." *Pastoral Care in Education* 27 (4):279-290.

Wylie, John. 2010. "Non-representational subjects." In *Taking-place: Non-representational Theories and Geography*, edited by Ben Anderson and Paul Harrison, 99-114. Farnham: Ashgate.

Yaneva, Albena. 2005. "Scaling up and down extraction trials in architectural design." *Social Studies of Science* 35 (6):867-894.

Yaneva, Albena. 2009a. *The Making of a Building: A Pragmatist Approach to Architecture*. Oxford: Peter Lang Publishers.

Yaneva, Albena. 2009b. "Making the social hold: Towards an Actor-Network Theory of design." *Design and Culture* 1 (3):273-288.

Yaneva, Albena. 2012. *Mapping Controversies in Architecture*. Farnham: Ashgate Publishing.

Yee, Donna L, John A Capitman, Walter N Leutz, and Mark Sceigaj. 1999. "Resident-centered care in assisted living." *Journal of Aging & Social Policy* 10 (3):7-26.

Youdell, Deborah. 2006. *Impossible Bodies, Impossible Selves: Exclusions and Student Subjectivities*. Vol. 3: Springer Science & Business Media.

Youdell, Deborah. 2011. *School Trouble: Identity, Power and Politics in Education*. Abington: Routledge.

Zimmerman, Sheryl, and Philip D Sloane. 2007. "Definition and classification of assisted living." *The Gerontologist* 47 (suppl 1):33-39.

Zimring, Craig. 1990. *The Costs of Confusion: Non-monetary and Monetary Costs of the Emory University Hospital Wayfinding System*. Atlanta: Georgia Institute of Technology.